Oxford Handbook of
Cardiac Nursing

Second Edition

Edited by

Kate Olson

Visiting Lecturer
City University
London
UK
and
Health Professional
Milton Keynes Community Cardiac Group
Milton Keynes
UK

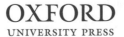

OXFORD
UNIVERSITY PRESS

OXFORD
UNIVERSITY PRESS

Great Clarendon Street, Oxford, OX2 6DP,
United Kingdom

Oxford University Press is a department of the University of Oxford.
It furthers the University's objective of excellence in research, scholarship,
and education by publishing worldwide. Oxford is a registered trade mark of
Oxford University Press in the UK and in certain other countries

First Edition published in 2007
Second Edition published in 2014

Impression: 1

Published in the United States of America by Oxford University Press
198 Madison Avenue, New York, NY 10016, United States of America

British Library Cataloguing in Publication Data
Data available

Library of Congress Control Number: 2013940285

ISBN 978-0-19-965134-4

Printed in China by
C&C Offset Printing Co. Ltd.

26.99

OXFORD MEDICAL PUBLICATIONS

Oxford Handbook of
Cardiac Nursing

Published and forthcoming Oxford Handbooks in Nursing

This book is dedicated to the memory of Shaun Bowden,
who contributed to the first edition of this book. Shaun was a loving
husband, dedicated dad to Isla and Callum, a great son, brother,
friend, and colleague and is missed by all who knew him

Foreword to second edition

Cardiac nursing is a wonderful speciality in which to work: it is interesting, dynamic, and challenging. Developments are made all the time in diagnostic and treatment techniques, and together with the increasing technology we now use, nurses have to be up to date, change their roles, be flexible, and combine well the technical and caring aspects of nursing. Most importantly, patients require care, understanding, and compassion and must be the focus of everything we do. Their needs and experiences of treatment and care are paramount and the priority placed on clinical effectiveness, patient safety, and an excellent patient experience helps provide a framework of good care.

Every day nurses interact with patients with cardiac problems in all healthcare settings. Some of this is acute, for example, the person who has a primary percutaneous angioplasty, however, much is chronic, such as for the person who has heart failure and has reached the time when end of life care is needed. The very young and the elderly, people with other physical and mental health problems alongside heart disease, men and women from different nationalities and backgrounds are all cared for by nurses in homes, clinics, and hospitals.

Being diagnosed with a cardiac problem will be stressful and raises many concerns for patients and their families. The implications of the diagnosis on quality and length of life, as well as for treatment and care, will be wide ranging and complex and may not be understood by the patient and family. Contrast the pattern of treatment for conditions such as an arrhythmia, infective endocarditis, or valvular disease: nurses have a role in helping patients with any of these. And there are risks associated with most interventions and nurses need to remember the vulnerability and fear felt in the face of decisions about surgery, insertion of devices, long-term drug therapy, and so on. We are increasingly aware of the implications, both positive and negative, of invasive interventions such as ventricular assist devices (VADs) and implantable cardiac defibrillators (ICDs). Each person deals with their anxiety and need for understanding in their own way and every nurse has to manage care to meet those needs.

This updated book gives a wealth of information in the technical elements of cardiac nursing. Reflecting the enormous changes that have taken place the book has been extensively revised to bring in the most up-to-date information. There are new sections on heart disease in pregnancy, congenital heart disease, and pulmonary artery hypertension. Risk factors and models of behaviour change have been included as well as standards on rehabilitation and the latest algorithms for resuscitation. Each chapter has related guidance from NICE, SIGN, the European Society of Cardiology, and the Cochrane Collaboration. It is a fantastic resource for the clinical nurse.

However, there will be more changes, some almost as soon as this book is published, so I encourage all nurses to read widely and keep alert to developments in this specialist field in order that each and every one can provide the best, most appropriate care to patients and their families.

Dr Caroline Shuldham OBE
Director of Nursing and
Clinical Governance
Royal Brompton and Harefield
NHS Foundation Trust
England

Foreword to first edition

Profound change in how and where cardiac care is delivered has occurred in the past six years since the National Service Framework (NSF) for Coronary Heart Disease (CHD) was published. The pace of change has been rapid in terms of both clinical advances and different service models for delivery of care. Cardiac nurses now move seamlessly across organisational boundaries, moving from a patient's home, to the GP practice and acute trust settings. This kind of increased movement across organizational boundaries means cardiac nurses require access to quick, portable, accessible information on the move; this new book will meet this need very well.

Cardiovascular disease is the United Kingdom's biggest cause of premature death and coronary heart disease accounts for more than 110,000 deaths in England each year. In March 2000, when the NSF for CHD was published, the early chapters focused on CHD patient pathways, but recently two new important documents have been published. The first in March 2005, a final chapter (Chapter 8) was added on Arrhythmia and Sudden Cardiac Death. This focused on the care of patients living with heart rhythm problems and families where a sudden cardiac death in the family has occurred. In May 2006, national commissioning guidance was published on the care of adolescents and adults with congenital heart disease. Many specialist cardiac nurses contributed to both these pieces of work, but not all cardiac nurses will have all the knowledge required. Both these areas are very well discussed in this new publication.

The Healthcare Commission, when reviewing progress on the implementation of the NSF for CHD, noted significant progress in access to early diagnosis, treatment of heart attack, and revascularization. In all these areas, cardiac nurses have made significant contributions. The Healthcare Commission also highlighted areas that require improvement, namely primary prevention, cardiac rehabilitation, and heart failure. A new government target is focusing on ensuring that, by 2008, no patient waits longer than 18 weeks from GP referral to treatment. This will increase the attention paid to diagnostic testing in cardiac care and I was delighted to see this book provides good descriptions of the common diagnostic tests as well as information on the three areas identified as needing improvement.

The editors, Kate Johnson and Karen Rawlings-Anderson, have created an excellent quick reference resource that will be a valuable addition to the Oxford Handbook series. It will be of great use where nurses deliver cardiac care, from work in primary care cardiovascular clinics to nurses working in the intensive care unit. In addition, I am sure it will be of value to the wider range of healthcare professionals and associates.

It will be a very welcome addition to libraries, the ward, or general practice, but especially for the nurse on the move.

Maree Barnett RN MSc MBA
Deputy Branch Head/Nurse Advisor
Vascular Programme
Department of Health
England

Preface to second edition

Since the publication of the first edition of the *Oxford Handbook of Cardiac Nursing* there have been a number of changes in the field of cardiac care. These changes have affected nurses working with cardiac patients in all different settings in both hospitals and the community. This edition has been completely revised and updated to reflect these changes. Each chapter now contains a list of relevant evidence-based guidelines from organizations such as the European Society of Cardiology and the National Institute for Health and Clinical Excellence. There is also a new section on heart disease in pregnancy. The chapter on congenital heart disease has been expanded and now contains information on pulmonary arterial hypertension. New pathways for the management of stable angina and for cardiac rehabilitation have been included as well as up-to-date resuscitation guidelines. The identification and management of risk factors has been addressed in more detail than before.

The feedback for the first edition of this book was very useful and has helped shape some of the changes for this edition. Feedback from readers for improvements for further editions would be welcome.

Kate Olson (née Johnson)
December 2012

Acknowledgements

I would like to thank everyone who has contributed to the development of this book. I would particularly like to thank the chapter contributors; Dr Caroline Shuldham, Kathryn Farrow, Anne Mcleod, and George O'Neill for their advice and feedback; and the reviewers who gave me useful and constructive feedback. I would also like to thank Karen Rawlings-Anderson who encouraged me to edit the first edition with her and for all her work on that edition.

I will be forever grateful to my family: Steve, Sophie, Sam, and Evie Olson who gave me unending support, patience, and understanding during the writing of this edition. My parents Roy and Maureen Thurkettle also deserve a mention for all their encouragement and support over the years.

Kate Olson
December 2012

Preface to first edition

Over the course of our nursing careers, we have both had times when we have been working in the clinical area and needed a cardiac reference text to hand. Whilst there are many excellent cardiac nursing textbooks available, in the clinical area nurses do not always have the time to read pages of detailed text. There did not seem to be a simple handbook on the market so we decided to write one!

This book gives an overview of cardiac nursing and is not intended to be a specialist text. Whilst we have touched on many specialist cardiac topics these have not all been covered in great depth (e.g. cardiac transplantation). The book takes the reader systematically from assessment through to investigation and treatment for a range of cardiac problems. This book will provide a handy reference for the nurse 'on the go' who wants a summary of the relevant issues related to their patients and the appropriate care required. Although primarily aimed at nurses working in cardiac practice, this book will also be invaluable for those working in other specialities who may care for patients who have cardiac problems.

Cardiac care is changing rapidly and we have tried to include principles of clinical management and give up-to-date information. We would welcome feedback from any reader who has suggestions for improvement for subsequent editions.

Kate Olson (née Johnson)
Karen Rawlings-Anderson
June 2007

Contents

Contributors to first edition

Shaun Bowden
Chapter 13
UK Account Manager
Hansen Medical

Lynda Filer
Chapter 19
Lecturer in Applied Biological
Sciences
St Bartholomew School of
Nursing and Midwifery
City University
London

Tracey Gibson
Chapter 8
Lecturer in Adult Nursing
St Bartholomew School of
Nursing and Midwifery
City University
London

Rachel Grant
Parts of Chapters 2 and 11
Lecturer in Critical Care Nursing
St Bartholomew School of
Nursing and Midwifery
City University
London

Sarah E Green
Chapters 7 and 15
Ward Sister
Coronary Care Unit
United Bristol Healthcare NHS
Trust
Bristol

Contributors to second edition

Tracey Bowden
Chapters 3, 7, and 8
Senior Lecturer in Cardiac Care
School of Health Sciences
City University
London, UK

Jane Butler
Chapters 10 and 15
Consultant Nurse
Barts Health NHS Trust
London Chest Hospital, UK

Lynda Filer
Chapter 19
Lecturer in Applied Biological
Sciences
School of Health Sciences
City University
London, UK

Rachel Grant
Chapters 2 and 11
Lecturer in Critical Care Nursing
School of Health Sciences
City University
London, UK

Shawn Holden
Chapter 13
Chief Cardiac Physiologist
St Bartholomew's Hospital
London, UK

Symbols and abbreviations

1°	primary
2°	secondary
▶	important
📖	cross reference
×	controversial topic
❶	warning
>	greater than
<	less than
♂	male
♀	female
∴	therefore
~	approximately
🖱	website
↑	increased/increasing
↓	decreased/decreasing
2D	two-dimensional
3D	three-dimensional
ABG	arterial blood gases
ABPM	ambulatory blood pressure monitoring
AC	atrial conduction
ACE	angiotensin-converting enzyme
ACHD	adult congenital heart disease
ACS	acute coronary syndromes
ACT	activated clotting time
ADH	antidiuretic hormone
ADP	adenosine diphosphate
A&E	Accident and Emergency Department
AECG	ambulatory electrocardiography monitoring
AED	automated external defibrillator
AF	atrial fibrillation
AH	atrium to His
ALS	advanced life support
AP	action potential
APPT	activated partial thromboplastin time
AR	aortic regurgitation

ARB	angiotensin receptor blockers
ARVC	arrhythmogenic right ventricular cardiomyopathy
AS	aortic stenosis
ASAP	as soon as possible
ASD	atrial septal defect
ASH	asymmetrical septal hypertrophy
AV	atrioventricular
AVNRT	atrioventricular node re-entry tachycardia
AVRT	atrioventricular re-entry tachycardia
AVPU	alert/voice/pain/unresponsive
AVR	aortic valve replacement
BBB	bundle branch block
BPM	beats per minute
BCL	basic cycle length
BE	base excess
BiPAP	bilevel positive airway pressure
BiVAD	biventricular assist device
BLS	basic life support
BMI	body mass index
BNP	B-type natriuretic peptide
BP	blood pressure
BVP	biventricular pacing
CABG	coronary artery bypass graft/s
CAD	coronary artery disease
CBT	cognitive behaviour therapy
CCF	congestive cardiac failure
CCU	Coronary Care Unit
CHB	complete heart block
CHD	coronary heart disease
CHF	chronic heart failure
CK	creatine kinase
CKD	chronic kidney disease
CK-MB	creatine kinase muscle and brain
CMR	cardiac magnetic resonance
CO	cardiac output
CO_2	carbon dioxide
COA	coarctation of the aorta
COPD	chronic obstructive pulmonary disease
CPAP	continuous positive airway pressure
CPB	cardiopulmonary bypass

CPR	cardiopulmonary resuscitation
CR	cardiac rehabilitation
CRT	capillary refill time or cardiac re-synchronization therapy
CS	coronary sinus
CSM	carotid sinus massage
CT	computed tomography
CVA	cerebrovascular accident
CVD	cardiovascular disease
CVP	central venous pressure
CVS	cardiovascular system
CWS	colour, warmth, sensation
CXR	chest X-ray
DCM	dilated cardiomyopathy
DC	direct current
DCT	distal convoluted tubule
DES	drug eluting stents
DKA	diabetic ketoacidosis
DN	district nurse
DVLA	Driver and Vehicle Licensing Authority
DVT	deep vein thrombosis
ECG	electrocardiogram
Echo	echocardiograph
ECMO	extra corporeal membrane oxygenation
EF	ejection fraction
EGM	electrogram
EHRA	European Heart Rhythm Association
EP	electrophysiology
EPS	electrophysiological study
ESC	European Society of Cardiology
ESR	erythrocyte sedimentation rate
ETT	exercise tolerance test
FAST	facial weakness, arm weakness, speech problems
FBC	full blood count
FH	familial hypercholesterolaemia
GFR	glomerular filtration rate
GI	gastrointestinal
GP	general practitioner
GTN	glyceryl trinitrate
GUCH	grown-up congenital heart [disease]
H_2O	water

Hb	haemoglobin
HCM	hypertrophic cardiomyopathy
HCO3	bicarbonate
HDL	high-density lipoprotein
HDU	high dependency unit
HFPEF	heart failure with preserved ejection fraction
Hg	mercury
HIV	human immunodeficiency virus
HMG-CoA	3-hydroxy-3-methyglutaryl-coenzyme A
HR	heart rate
HRA	high right atrium
HV	His to ventricle interval
IABP	intra-aortic balloon pump
IACT	intra-atrial conduction time
ICD	implantable cardioverter-defibrillator
ICP	intra cranial pressure
IE	infective endocarditis
IM	intramuscular
IMA	internal mammary artery
INR	international normalized ratio
ITU	Intensive Therapy Unit
IV	intravenous
JVP	jugular venous pressure
K^+	potassium
LA	left atrium/atrial
LAD	left anterior descending
LAH	left atrial hypertrophy
LBBB	left bundle branch block
LDL	low-density lipoprotein
LFT	liver function test
LGV	large goods vehicle
LMS	left main stem
LMWH	low-molecular-weight heparin
LV	left ventricle/ventricular
LVAD	left ventricular assist device
LVEDP	left ventricular end diastolic pressure
LVEF	left ventricular ejection fraction
LVF	left ventricular failure
LVH	left ventricular hypertrophy
LVOT	left ventricular outflow tract

LVOTO	left ventricular outflow tract obstruction
LVSD	left ventricular systolic dysfunction
MAP	mean arterial pressure
M,C&S	microscopy, sensitivity, & culture
MI	myocardial infarction
MIDCAB	minimally invasive direct coronary artery bypass
MPS	myocardial perfusion scintigraphy
MR	mitral regurgitation
MRI	magnetic resonance imaging
MRSA	meticillin resistant *Staphylococcus aureus*
MS	mitral stenosis
MUGA	multiple gated acquisition
MV	mitral valve
MVP	mitral valve prolapse
MVR	mitral valve replacement
Na$^+$	sodium
NAC	N-acetylcysteine
NaCl	sodium chloride
NACR	National Audit for Cardiac Rehabilitation
NG	nasogastric
NHS	National Health Service
NICE	National Institute for Health and Care Excellence
NIV	noninvasive ventilation
NMS	neurally mediated syncope
NRT	nicotine replacement therapy
NSAID	nonsteroidal anti-inflammatory drug
NSF	National Service Framework
NSTEMI	non-ST segment elevation myocardial infarction
NVE	native valve endocarditis
NYHA	New York Heart Association
O2	oxygen
PA	pulmonary artery
PAH	pulmonary arterial hypertension
PAP	pulmonary artery pressure
PAWP	pulmonary artery wedge pressure
PCA	patient controlled analgesia
PCI	percutaneous coronary intervention
PCT	proximal convoluted tubule
PCV	packed cell volume
PDA	patent ductus arteriosus

PE	pulmonary embolism
PEA	pulseless electrical activity
PEEP	positive end expiratory pressure
PES	programmed electrical stimulation
PET	positron emission tomography
PFO	patent foramen ovale
PND	paroxysmal nocturnal dyspnoea
PoTs	postural orthostatic tachycardia syndrome
PPCI	primary percutaneous coronary intervention
PPM	permanent pacemaker
PS	pulmonary stenosis
PSV	passenger service vehicle
PTCA	percutaneous transluminal coronary angioplasty
PTT	partial thromboplastin time
PVD	peripheral vascular disease
PVE	prosthetic valve endocarditis
PVR	pulmonary vascular resistance
RA	right atrium/atrial
RAAS	renin–angiotensin–aldosterone system
RAH	right atrial hypertrophy
RBBB	right bundle branch block
RCM	restrictive cardiomyopathy
RFA	radiofrequency ablation
RR	respiratory rate
RSVP	reason, story, vital signs, plan
RV	right ventricle/ventricular
RVA	right ventricular apex
RVAD	right ventricular assist device
RVF	right ventricular failure
RVH	right ventricular hypertrophy
RVOT	right ventricular outflow tract
RVOTO	right ventricular outflow tract obstruction
SA	sino-atrial
SaO2	oxygen saturation
SAECG	signal average ECG
SBAR	situation, background, assessment, recommendation
SC	subcutaneous
SCD	sudden cardiac death
SIGN	Scottish Intercollegiate Guidelines Network
SIMV	spontaneous intermittent mandatory ventilation

S/L	sub-lingual
SLE	systemic lupus erythematosus
SNP	serum natriuretic peptides
SOB	shortness of breath
SOBOE	shortness of breath on exertion
SPECT	single photon emission computerized tomography
SpO$_2$	peripheral oxygen saturation
STEMI	ST-segment elevation myocardial infarction
SV	stroke volume
SVE	supraventricular ectopic
SVT	supraventricular tachycardia
TAVI	transcatheter aortic valve implantation
TAVR	transcatheter aortic valve implantation
TFT	thyroid function test
TGA	transposition of the great arteries
TIA	transient ischaemic attack
TLoC	transient loss of consciousness
TOE	transoesophageal echocardiograph
TOF	tetralogy of Fallot
TS	tricuspid stenosis
TTE	transthoracic echocardiograph
U&E	urea & electrolytes
UA	unstable angina
UK	United Kingdom
UTI	urinary tract infection
VA	venoarterial
VAD	venticular assist device
VE	ventricular ectopic
VF	ventricular fibrillation
VSD	ventricular septal defect
VT	ventricular tachycardia
VTE	venous thromboembolism
VV	venovenous
WBC	white blood cell
WPW	Wolff–Parkinson–White
Yrs	years

Introduction: prevention of cardiovascular disease

What does the book cover?

This book is intended as a quick reference for nurses working in areas where they care for patients with cardiac problems. It does not cover every aspect of cardiac disease in great depth but provides the essential information required to care for patients presenting with cardiac problems. Although cardiovascular disease (CVD) affects the entire cardiovascular system, the scope of this book does not enable discussion of peripheral vascular disease (PVD) and stroke but focuses on cardiac disease and its management. This book covers all the forms of heart disease that nurses working in the cardiac field might encounter (e.g. valvular disease, infective diseases, congenital and inherited diseases of the heart, common arrhythmias, and cardiac emergencies), but the primary focus is on coronary heart disease (CHD), which remains one of the largest single killers in the UK. Related topics are cross-referenced within the book where relevant.

The book covers a wide range of issues pertinent to nursing patients with cardiac problems irrespective of the clinical arena in which they are managed. The initial chapters of the book cover the assessment of the patient and outline the investigations that the patient might have. Interventions that the patient might require and pharmacological management are also included.

The book gives relevant information to nurses working in a variety of specialities in the UK. Patients with cardiac problems are not always managed in a specialist unit; indeed, many of those with cardiac disease present with their first symptoms to a general practitioner (GP) or practice nurse, or their symptoms are picked up when they are treated for another, unrelated problem. Whether you work in primary care, a general ward, or within a specialist cardiac service this book will help you find out about the essential elements of cardiac problems that you might not be familiar with. For more in-depth information on specific topics, there are a variety of texts and journals readily available on the market. Each chapter has a list of appropriate guidelines at the end of the chapter and suggested further reading and resources can also be found at the end of the book in the Appendix.

This introductory chapter briefly outlines the context within which cardiac care exists. It identifies the extent of the burden of cardiac disease and the background of policy drivers that have influenced recent developments in cardiac care. A discussion of the risk factors for CVD and health promotion is also included.

Mortality and morbidity

CVD is the main cause of death in the UK, accounting for >180 000 deaths in 2009. Of all deaths from CVD, ~49% are from CHD and >27% are from stroke. Over one and half million people living in the UK have had a heart attack and over 2million have angina and/or heart failure.[1]

Since the 1960s the death rate from CVD in the UK has been falling and CVD has now been overtaken by cancer as the most common cause of premature death (before the age of 75) in the UK.[1] Despite this, CHD mortality rates have remained 30–40% higher in Scotland than England since 1961.

With the advent of antibiotic therapy, the prevalence of valvular heart disease related to rheumatic fever has ↓. Moreover, those born with congenital heart defects are now surviving because of advances in surgical techniques and the life expectancy of those born with congenital heart defects has ↑ considerably since the 1960s. The number of patients surviving acute cardiac events, such as myocardial infarction (MI), is also ↑; however, this has led to an ↑ number of patients who later go on to develop chronic heart failure (CHF). While smoking rates have been falling the rates of obesity and diabetes have ↑ which may lead to a reversal in trends in the future if not appropriately addressed. Thus, it can be seen that cardiac care has had to change considerably in the last decade or so to meet the needs of the ever-changing population of patients with cardiac problems.

[1] British Heart Foundation (2011) Trends in Coronary Heart Disease 1961–2011. British Heart Foundation, London.

Policy context

In the last decade a number of national evidence-based standards and guidelines for CVD have been instigated across the UK. In 2000 the publication of the *National Service Framework for Coronary Heart Disease*[2] (NSF for CHD) in England imposed targets in 12 areas related to CHD, ranging from 1° prevention and 2° prevention to diagnosis, management, and rehabilitation for those with CHD. The NSF targets influenced the development of new and improved services for those with CHD, and a new chapter relating to arrhythmias and sudden cardiac death was subsequently published to supplement the original targets.[3]

The Heart Disease and Stroke Strategy for Scotland published in 2002 was revised in 2009[4] and the *The Cardiac Disease National Service Framework for Wales*,[5] was published in 2009 to update the original Welsh NSF for CHD published in 2002.

While many of the original NSF targets were achieved and in some cases exceeded this was not the case for all areas, e.g. cardiac rehabilitation. This is now one of the priority areas for NHS Improvement Heart.[6] Others include:
- Atrial fibrillation (AF)
- Heart failure
- Reperfusion
- Cardiac surgery
- Arrhythmia and sudden cardiac death
- NHS Health Check
- Stroke Improvement Programme.

The implementation of these priority areas in England is through the work of 28 cardiac networks that also share best practice and provide a source of information and support.

A number of evidence-based guidelines have also been published by organizations such as the National Institute for Health and Care Excellence (NICE), Scottish Intercollegiate Guidelines Network (SIGN), and European Society of Cardiology (ESC) which help to streamline the care of patients with CVD and ensure that clinical decision-making and management of the patient's condition is based on the best available evidence.

Non-governmental organizations such as the National Heart Forum (⌂ http://www.heartforum.org.uk), European Heart Network (⌂ http://www.ehnheart.org), and the World Heart Federation (⌂ http://www.world-heart-federation.org) work to influence policy-making in CVD prevention and will often advise Governments on policies and strategies for CVD. They are made up of a number of other organizations including charities and consumer groups. There are also a number of groups that are responsible for auditing cardiac services throughout the UK.

CVD is a major public health issue, resulting in the prevention, diagnosis, and management of CHD moving beyond traditional tertiary specialist services and becoming the province of healthcare professionals in both 1° care and 2° care. Patients with cardiac disease are cared for in a wide range of areas.

Overall, the last 10–15yrs have shown significant policy initiatives within the UK in relation to the diagnosis, management, and prevention of cardiac disease. These, alongside technological advances, have meant considerable developments in the care and management of people with cardiac problems. Patient choice and the introduction of the 18wk referral to treatment have meant that not only do patients have more choice as to where they get their treatment but they also wait less time than in previous years. This has had a big impact on how services are designed with many being redesigned to accommodate this.

[2] Department of Health (2000) *The National Service Framework for Coronary Heart Disease*. DH, London.

[3] Department of Health (2005) Arrhythmias and sudden cardiac death. Chapter 8 in *National Service Framework for Coronary Heart Disease*. DH, London.

[4] NHS Scotland (2009) *Better Heart Disease and Stroke Care Action Plan*. The Scottish Government, Edinburgh.

[5] Welsh Assembly Government (2009) *The Cardiac Disease National Service Framework for Wales*. WAG, Cardiff

[6] NHS Improvement Heart: http://www.improvment/nhs/uk/heart

Cardiac developments and trends

Healthcare is ever changing. Nurses are used to working in an environment where research, policies, targets, audit data, and guidelines amongst other things, all influence and change the nature of day-to-day work. In 2013, plans regarding urgent care have been put in place, the Cardiovascular Disease Outcomes Strategy has been published by the Department of Health, and a new vision for nursing and midwifery has also been shared. Each of these has an impact on cardiac nursing. Other areas that continue to shape cardiac care are highlighted here.

Technology

Technology has been used in a number of ways in healthcare for many years. However, in the last few years we have seen a growth in areas such as telehealth which has been particularly useful in the care of patients with long-term conditions. Research comparing patients receiving telemonitoring compared to usual care found ↓ hospital admissions, ↓ mortality rates and ↓ visits to emergency departments.[7] Other areas where technology is being used are as follows:

- Virtual wards—where patients are in their homes but are linked to a hospital setting
- Remote monitoring, e.g. blood pressure (BP), remote monitoring of devices
- Electronic records
- Use of laptops, tablets, and other devices for those working in the community to avoid having to keep returning to a central base
- Use of websites, mobile apps, blogs, online communities, forums, Quick Response (QR) codes, and other Internet sources for information for patients and health professionals
- New technology for procedures, e.g. robotics
- Use of text messaging to support and contact patients
- Use of social media such as Twitter for information sharing and support.

Each of these areas brings opportunities and challenges. Some are already commonplace and it is important that through organizations such as the cardiac networks that good practice is shared. Resistance to using technology may come from both patients and staff and so it is important that strategies are put into place to ensure that people understand the reason for the technology and the benefits of using it. While some patients will enjoy the benefits of being monitored in their own home, for others this can make them feel anxious and possibly isolated. Any sources of information used should be evidence based and professional guidelines relating to social media and the like must be adhered to.

Organization of care and nursing roles

Since the advent of 1° percutaneous coronary intervention (PPCI) as the 'gold standard' for treating ST-segment elevation myocardial infarction (STEMI), care of patients has moved away from traditional Coronary Care Units (CCUs) to 'Heart Attack Centres'. This has meant that many CCUs now have a very different patient profile than previously. Some units now take patients with other medical conditions warranting acute care, whereas other units have specialized in an area of cardiac care such as electrophysiology. This naturally has an impact on the nursing staff with some having to become more generalized in their knowledge base whereas others have had to develop a more specific focus.

A report published in 2011[8] suggested that CCUs should be renamed Acute Cardiac Units under the care of a cardiologist and with access to key investigations. The types of patients that should be admitted would be those with non-ST-segment elevation myocardial infarction (NSTEMI) or unstable angina (UA), acute decompensating heart failure, narrow and broad tachycardias, symptomatic bradycardia, pulmonary embolism (PE), infective endocarditis (IE), pericardial effusion, cardiac device management, and acute thoracic emergencies such as aortic dissection.

Other changes in treatments such as transcatheter aortic valve implantation (TAVI) for valve replacement have also led to changes in the way care is organized and the types of clinical areas that patients go to. Hospital length of stay has been ↓ in some cases with hospital at home schemes or telemonitoring put in place so that patients can return home sooner.

Many patients will be managed by a team of people that will be made up of a number of different health professionals such as cardiac physiologists, physiotherapists, and nurse specialists. This is particularly the case with conditions such as heart failure and those with device implantations. In some cases new roles have come into existence such as physician's assistants and perioperative specialist practitioners. Many of these services are nurse-led with nurses taking over many of the roles previously performed by doctors. There are also more examples of nurses working in collaboration with the users of healthcare to ensure services meet the patients' needs.

Research and development

Research into CVD is ongoing and constantly informs the work of health professionals. This might be the development of new procedures, evidence of better outcomes with certain medications, or breakthroughs in scientific discoveries, particularly in the field of genetics and stem cell research. Whilst not all nurses will be involved in undertaking research each has the opportunity to ensure they keep up to date with current evidence-based practice.

[7] ℘ http://http://3millionlives.co.uk

[8] British Cardiovascular Society (2011) *From Coronary Care Unit to Acute Cardiac Care Unit – the evolving role of specialist cardiac care.* BSC, London.

Prevention of cardiovascular disease

A number of national and European guidelines have been published that relate to the prevention of CVD, some of which are listed at the end of this chapter (🕮 Related guidance, p.23). Prevention may be 1° (for those without established disease) or 2° (those with established disease). The two main approaches that are used are either the population approach, which may target everyone through areas such as policy, legislation, transport, food industry, to make healthy choices easier choices or a high-risk approach. This targets interventions at those who already have established disease or who have a high risk of developing a disease. Usually a combination of both approaches will be recommended.

It is important that messages regarding healthy behaviours are given throughout the lifespan, particularly as levels of childhood obesity are ↑. Evidence suggests that there should not be an upper age limit as older people can benefit from making positive changes to their health. Recent NICE guidance on the prevention of CVD at population level[9] suggested a number of recommendations which addresses issues such as salt consumption, the marketing of unhealthy food to children and young people, food labelling, reduction of trans fats, and schemes for active forms of transport.

NHS Health Check

Health checks (originally known as vascular checks) are available in England to all those aged between 40–74 who do not already have a diagnosis of vascular disease.[10] There are similar programmes in Wales and Scotland. A risk assessment (🕮 Risk factor assessment, p.9) will be carried out looking at a number of factors using questions, measurements, and blood tests. From this information a patient may be categorized according to their risk of developing CVD and given appropriate advice and, if necessary, further treatment.

---

[9] National Institute for Health and Clinical Excellence (2010) *Prevention of Cardiovascular Disease at Population Level*. NICE, London. 🕭 http://www.nice.org.uk

[10] Department of Health (2009) *NHS Health Check: Vascular Risk Assessment and Management Best Practice Guidance*. The Stationery Office, London.

Risk factors for cardiovascular disease

The risk factors discussed here are mainly for CVD. Although there does not seem to be one single risk factor that causes CVD, it has been established that those who develop CVD will usually have a combination of risk factors. Risk factors are divided into nonmodifiable, modifiable, behavioural, and psychosocial factors (Table 1.1). The ones discussed in this chapter are those that have been clearly established to ↑ the risk of CVD.

A number of other factors might also ↑ the risk for CVD. These include the following:

• Low birth weight
• Inflammatory markers, such as plasma C-reactive protein
• Thrombogenic factors such as homocysteine
• Platelet-activating factors
• Other conditions such as erectile dysfunction and obstructive sleep apnoea.

The effects of these factors are the subject of ongoing research and they are, as yet, not fully established as risk factors, so will not be discussed here.

Risk factor assessment

Risk factor assessment usually takes place in 1° care and might be performed in a nurse-led risk factor prevention clinic. Although CVD prevention should focus on people with established disease, those with diabetes or those at high risk (CVD risk >20% over 10yrs), it is now recommended that all people aged 40–74yrs have a risk factor assessment. This should include questions about smoking history, family history of CVD, and measurement of BP; blood tests for glucose levels and total cholesterol, high- (HDL) and low-density lipoprotein (LDL); weight, and waist circumference; in addition to an assessment of lifestyle factors, such as physical activity levels. Many risk factor scoring tools can then be used to predict an individual's risk of developing CVD. When calculating this risk, consider a prior history of diabetes, medication, organ damage, CVD, and ethnicity. Tools that may be used include SCORE,[11] ASSIGN,[12] or QRisk.[13] It is important to remember that while a young person with several risk factors may have a fairly low absolute risk of developing CVD their relative risk compared to someone of the same age without those risk factors will be high. A number of tools will also have algorithms for treatment management. Audit risk factors regularly.

Table 1.1 Risk factors for CVD

Nonmodifiable	Modifiable	Behavioural	Psychosocial
• Age	• Hypertension	• Smoking	• Stress
• ♂ gender	• Renal disease	• Low levels of physical activity	• Low socio-economic status
• Family history	• Dietary factors (e.g. ↑ cholesterol and ↑ triglycerides)	• ↑ Alcohol	• Social isolation
• Ethnicity			• Depression
• Premature menopause	• ↑ waist circumference		• ↑ Anxiety, hostility, or anger
	• Insulin resistance		

Nonmodifiable risk factors

Age

The development of atherosclerosis takes place over a number of years and, ∴, the risk of developing CHD ↑ with age, particularly over the age of 65yrs. Individuals might have also developed other comorbidities, such as diabetes and hypertension, which are both independent risk factors for CVD.

Ethnicity

↑ levels of CVD are seen in the South East Asian population (~1.4 times higher than predicted for the rest of the population). This is often associated with higher levels of diabetes, familial hypercholesterolaemia (FH), and ↑ waist circumference. Although individuals from Africa and the Caribbean have a lower level of CHD, they have higher levels of hypertension and stroke.

Gender

♂ have higher rates of CHD because of the protective effects of oestrogen in ♀ before the menopause. Over the age of 75yrs the rates are equal. ♀ often present later and frequently have atypical symptoms; coronary arteries are smaller in ♀ and they are more likely to suffer with Syndrome X (☐ Syndrome X, p.112). They also seem to have more severe complications following MI and surgery.

Family history

A family history of CHD is considered a risk factor. The risk is ↑ for the following reasons:
• CHD in a close family member—e.g. sibling or parent
• Number of relatives with CHD
• The age at which CHD first presented—the younger the presentation, the greater the risk.

In some cases, there could be a history of FH. If this is the case, it is important that all family members are regularly screened. Family history also has an important role in cardiac diseases that have genetic links, such as cardiomyopathy.

Modifiable risk factors: 1

Smoking

Smoking causes a number of diseases, including many cancers. The risks associated with CVD are attributable to the chemicals within cigarettes. Some of these have an effect on the endothelium and ↑ the likelihood of atherosclerosis developing. Carbon monoxide binds more readily with haemoglobin than oxygen (O_2) and, ∴, ↓ the amount of O_2 available to the myocardium. Nicotine leads to the release of adrenaline, which causes vasoconstriction and, ∴, ↑ the workload of the heart. It also leads to hypertension and ↑ platelet aggregation. The impact of smoking is greater on those with hypertension or diabetes.

Smoking cessation

When assessing smoking history, it is important to consider both the number of cigarettes smoked per day and the number of years the individual has smoked. This is also important in those who might have stopped smoking for a few years but who previously smoked for many years. Previous attempts at quitting and the methods used should also be assessed.

Strategies for smoking cessation include advice, nicotine-replacement therapy (NRT), and medication. Although individually each of these is proven to be successful, the strategy used should consider the individual's dependence on smoking and their motivation to quit. If they have a high motivation and low dependence, advice might be enough. If, however, they have a high dependence, they will probably require NRT. Referral to trained smoking cessation advisors should be offered.

Advice

Even brief advice (5min) can be successful, so it is important that healthcare professionals discuss smoking where possible. Health professionals are advised to use the 3 As[14]: Ask and record smoking status; Advise patients of health benefits of stopping; Act on patient's response.

Questions should focus on the individual's smoking habit, their dependence on smoking, their willingness to give up smoking, and their understanding of the effects smoking has on their health. Motivational interviewing (📖 Motivational interviewing, p.20) has proven to be beneficial in assisting with smoking cessation. Other patients may find Internet-based interventions useful such as ℅ http://www.smokefree.nhs.uk which has a number of tools to help people assess addiction and look at the method best suited to them to help them stop smoking.

NRT

NRT can take the form of gum, lozenges, microtabs, inhalators, nasal spray, and patches. The product used will depend on the patient's preference and advice of the clinician as some products may be contraindicated. NRT is beneficial for patients who have a high level of dependence on smoking.

Medication

Bupropion can decrease the desire to smoke and the withdrawal symptoms. It should be taken 1–2wks prior to quitting smoking. There are a number of contraindications such as pregnancy, breastfeeding, and a history of bipolar disorder. It should not be prescribed to under 18s. Side effects include seizure (rare), dry mouth, rash, and insomnia.

Varenicline has been specifically developed to help with smoking cessation. It also reduces the desire to smoke and ↓ withdrawal symptoms. It also has a number of contraindications such as pregnancy, breastfeeding and should be used with caution in those with psychiatric illness as it may ↑ suicidal thoughts. It should not be prescribed to under 18s.

Relapse

Although some patients can be successful in quitting at their first attempt, for others smoking cessation can take longer. If the patient does relapse, the nurse should help them to understand the reasons for this and encourage them to have another attempt at giving up smoking.

---

14 Department of Health (2009). *NHS Stop Smoking Services – Service and Monitoring Guidance 2009/10*. DH, London.

Modifiable risk factors: 2

Hypertension

High BP (systolic BP >140mmHg and diastolic BP >90mmHg) leads to ↑ cardiac workload and ↑ the risk of stroke, organ damage (e.g. renal impairment), and PVD. It can be caused by smoking, high sodium intake, and, to a certain extent, ↑ levels of stress over a period of time. However, in some cases there is no identifiable cause. This is known as 'essential hypertension'. NICE guidance on 1° hypertension[15] recommends that if a recorded BP is 140/90mmHg or above they should be offered ambulatory blood pressure monitoring (ABPM) to confirm diagnosis. Home monitoring can be used as an alternative.

Dietary modification, stopping smoking, and ↑ levels of physical activity all help to lower BP levels. Recommendations[15] for offering anti-hypertensive medication are as follows:

- Stage 1 hypertension—average BP >135/85mmHg, aged <80yrs with one of the following: CVD, target organ damage, renal disease, diabetes or 10yr CVD risk ≥20%
- Stage 2 hypertension—average measurement of ≥150/95mmHg at any age
- Those <40yrs with stage 1 hypertension but none of the factors listed here should be investigated for other 2° causes of hypertension.

Medication used may include calcium-channel blockers, angiotensin-converting enzyme (ACE) inhibitors, angiotensin II receptor blockers, or thiazide-like diuretic. The choice will depend on the patient's age, ethnicity, and the effectiveness of the medication.

Alcohol

Evidence seems to suggest that 1–3 units of alcohol (of any type) per day ↓ the risk of CHD. However, >3 units ↑ the risk, particularly in relation to ↑ triglycerides. Excessive alcohol consumption can also cause hypertension, some types of cardiomyopathy, rhythm abnormalities, and sudden cardiac death.

Psychosocial factors

Stress is often mentioned as a risk factor for CVD. However, for those without CVD, stress alone is unlikely to cause a problem and a certain level of stress can be beneficial. Stress can lead to the adoption of unhealthy behaviours, such as smoking, ↑ alcohol consumption, poor diet, and lack of physical activity. In those with established CHD, stress prior to a heart attack has been shown to ↑ platelet activation and lead to a slower recovery of normal BP following the event.

Low socioeconomic status, lack of social support, and ↑ depression, anxiety, and hostility may all contribute to the development of CVD and also contribute to a poor prognosis following a cardiac event. A psychosocial assessment should be conducted and, if necessary, the use of appropriate tools to help assess psychological state in more detail. Referral to appropriate services such as counselling, cognitive behavioural therapy (CBT), or other appropriate therapy may be required.

Physical activity

Lack of regular physical activity (aerobic activity) leads to an ↑ risk of CVD developing as well as contributing to obesity. Physical activity can lead to an ↑ of HDL, weight loss, ↓ risk of stroke, ↓ risk of developing diabetes, ↓ in BP, and improved cardiac function. Those that have been physically active are more likely to survive a heart attack than those that have not.

Recommendations[16] for physical activity suggest that healthy adults should undertake 2.5–5h of moderate intensity per week. This can be broken down into sessions to suit the individual. High-intensity interval training has been shown to be more beneficial than moderate-intensity continuous training.

Those with previous MI, coronary artery bypass graft (CABG), PCI, stable angina, or stable heart failure who have low clinical risk should be encouraged to do 30min at least 3×/week (broken into 10min segments if required). See the chapter on cardiac rehabilitation (Chapter 17) for further information on exercising post cardiac event.

[15] National Institute for Health and Clinical Excellence (2011) *Hypertension: Clinical Management of Primary Hypertension in Adults.* NICE, London. ✆ http://www.nice.org.uk

[16] Perk J, DeBacker G, Gohlke H, *et al.* for the Fifth Joint Task Force of the European Society of Cardiology and Other Societies on Cardiovascular Disease Prevention in Clinical Practice (2012) European Guidelines on cardiovascular disease prevention in clinical practice (version 2012). *European Heart Journal* **33**, 1635–701.

Dietary factors

Obesity

Obesity has been on the increase for several years. Of particular concern has been the ↑ in obesity in children and young adults. Obesity is a risk factor for CVD, type 2 diabetes, and stroke. Obesity may be caused by a combination of factors such as genetic, social, environmental, neuroendocrine, life stages, and life events such as pregnancy. Assessment should include blood tests to rule out metabolic causes such as an underactive thyroid. History of weight gain, any medications that may affect weight, current dietary and physical activity habits, and previous attempts to lose weight should all be assessed. Body mass index (BMI) and waist circumference should be recorded.

Waist circumference is felt to be a better predictor than BMI for CVD risk. Measure waist circumference midway between the lowest rib and the iliac crest while the patient is breathing out. A waist circumference >94cm in ♂ and >80cm in ♀ (>90cm in Asian men) is considered an ↑ risk for the development of both diabetes and CVD.

Weight management programmes should include dietary change, physical activity, and behavioural support and should be evidence based. In some cases pharmacological support such as orlistat may also be required. CBT and Motivational interviewing (📖 Motivational interviewing, p.20) have both been found to be useful approaches. A small regular weight loss over a period of time should be encouraged. It is important that the patient understands the reasons for their weight gain and sets realistic goals for themselves in order to achieve the desired weight loss.

School programmes and family-based lifestyle interventions have been suggested as ways of tackling obesity in children and young adults.

Cholesterol

↑ levels of cholesterol, particularly high levels of LDL, contribute to the development of atherosclerosis. It is important that total cholesterol, LDL, HDL, and triglycerides are all considered. ↑ levels of HDL help to remove excess cholesterol and, ∴, management of cholesterol should include ways of ↑ HDL. ↑ levels of triglycerides are also thought to lead to an ↑ risk of developing CVD, particularly in the presence of ↑ LDL and ↓ HDL. High levels of saturated fat in the diet lead to an ↑ in cholesterol, particularly LDL. Polyunsaturates help to ↑ the levels of HDL and thus ↓ cholesterol levels. Dietary cholesterol has very little impact on cholesterol levels. Targets for cholesterol in those at low or moderate risk of CVD are <5.0mmol/L for total cholesterol and <3.0mmol/L for LDL.[17] For those who are at high risk or very high CVD risk (based on SCORE risk) the targets for LDL are <2.5mmol/L and <1.8mmol/L respectively.

FH is an inherited disorder leading to very high cholesterol concentrations in the blood and ↑ incidence of premature CVD. A diagnosis of FH should be suspected in adults with total serum cholesterol >7.5mmol/L or an LDL level >5.2mmol/L and a family history of premature CVD.[18]

Statins

Although diet might help to ↓ total cholesterol in many patients, statins will also need to be prescribed (📖 Statins, p.379). NICE guidance[18] recommends that lipid-lowering therapy should be given to anyone with clinical evidence of CVD or as 1° prevention of CVD for adults who have a 20% or greater 10yr risk of developing CVD. Simvastatin or pravastatin are usually used. Liver function tests should be performed when treatment is started and at 3 and 12 months.

Diet

Dietary advice must be realistic, practical, and, if possible, tailored to the individual. The nurse should also take account of factors such as culture and religion. Involving other family members should be encouraged. In some instances, referral to a dietician might be required. If the patient has newly diagnosed diabetes mellitus, they should be referred to a nurse specialist in diabetes mellitus. General dietary guidelines for cardioprotection include the following:

• At least five portions of fruit and vegetable per day
• ↓ fat intake to <30% of total energy intake
• ↓ saturated fat intake to <10% of total fat intake (monounsaturated fat should be eaten instead)
• Sources of omega-3 fatty acids, e.g. fish, should be eaten twice weekly
• Limit salt intake
• 30–45g of fibre/day from wholegrains, fruit, vegetables
• Limit intake of processed food
• The recommended alcohol intake should be limited to 21–28 units/wk for ♂ or 14–21 units/wk for ♀. However, individuals should have set targets for cutting down, depending on their consumption.

It is also recommended that individuals should aim for a BMI of 20–25kg/m^2 and avoid central obesity.

[17] Reiner Z, Catapano A, deBacker G, et al. (2011) ESC/EAS guidelines for the management of dyslipidaemias. The Task Force on the management of dyslipidaemias of the European Society of Cardiology (ESC) and the European Atherosclerosis Society (EAS). European Heart Journal **32**, 1769–818.

[18] National Institute for Health and Clinical Excellence (2010) Lipid Modification: Cardiovascular Risk Assessment and the Modification of Blood Lipids for the Primary and Secondary Prevention of Cardiovascular Disease. NICE, London. ✍ http://www.nice.org.uk

Diabetes

There are currently ~1.8 million diagnosed diabetics in the UK, with many other individuals who have undiagnosed diabetes. This number is predicted to ↑ during the next few years. Patients with diabetes are ~2–4 times more likely to develop CVD than those without diabetes. ↑ insulin resistance leads to an ↑ in atheroma formation. A diagnosis of type 2 diabetes is made if the glycated haemoglobin (HBA₁c) is 6.5% (48mmol/mol) or above or a random venous plasma glucose of 11.1mmol or higher; or fasting glucose >7mmol/L. All diabetics should be treated aggressively for CVD prevention and would normally be prescribed a statin. Dietary advice and medication will be used (usually metformin) to help stabilize blood glucose levels and reduce risk.

Metabolic syndrome

The metabolic syndrome is a collection of factors that can help predict the risk of the development of type 2 diabetes mellitus and CVD. The metabolic syndrome is usually diagnosed if three or more of the following are present:

- Central obesity, as measured by waist circumference
- Triglyceride level >1.7mmol/L
- Low HDL levels—<1.0mmol/L in ♂ and <1.3mmol/L in ♀
- ↑ BP >135/85mmHg
- Fasting glucose >6.1mmol/L.

Behaviour change

Each individual has their own concept of health and what being healthy means, which usually involves a mixture of physical, emotional, social, spiritual, and psychological factors. These factors will vary in importance, depending on different situations, and definitions of health can change over time.

Health professionals need to be aware of how each individual defines health because this will help them target appropriate health-promotion interventions. The influence of values, attitudes, and beliefs must also be taken into consideration because these will influence how a patient feels about the maintenance of their health. For example, if a person believes that what happens to them is in the hands of fate (external locus of control), they are less likely to feel that they can influence the outcome by altering their behaviour. However, someone with a strong internal locus of control will feel that they can influence their life by the way they behave. Although it seems that those with an internal locus of control are more likely to accept advice regarding behaviour change, it does not always follow that they will adhere to it. It can also be difficult for patients with a strong internal locus of control to accept change if they have an MI despite having no obvious modifiable risk factors.

Nurses who are regularly working with patients on lifestyle management should ideally have training in motivational interviewing and relapse prevention strategies. Behaviour change is a combination of social, psychological, and environmental factors. An understanding of the stages of change model[19] can help when discussing risk factors with patients.

The stages of change model

The stages of change model[19] is particularly well known in relation to smoking cessation, although it can be applied to any behavioural change. The authors suggest that individuals normally go through a cycle of change before adopting more healthy behaviours. Although it is accepted that the person could relapse, it is suggested that the more times they go round the cycle, the more probable it is that they will achieve success. Individuals can stay at any individual stage for a length of time or might move quickly through the stages. The stages are as follows:

- Precontemplation—the person is not interested in changing their behaviour. At this stage, the health professional can ensure that the individual understands the risks of continuing with their actions.
- Contemplation—at this stage, the individual is thinking about changing and might be weighing-up the advantages and disadvantages of changing their behaviour. The health professional can help by getting the individual to think about the benefits of behaviour change.
- Ready for action—at this stage, the individual has decided to change their behaviour but might need assistance with deciding what intervention is needed to achieve this.
- Action—the individual has changed behaviour and will need support and encouragement to continue with the changed behaviour.
- Maintenance/relapsing—either could occur.

This model is particularly useful in helping health professionals to target their advice according to where the individual is in relation to the cycle.

Although models and theories might be useful, it is important to remember that behavioural change takes time, and although the process can start in hospital, it needs to be followed up once the patient returns home. Health promotion is most successful if it focuses on the needs and goals of the patient rather than those of the healthcare professional.

Motivational interviewing

The purpose of motivational interviewing[20] is to work with patients on goals that are important to them. The values and goals of the individual need to be established at the start and these are used as the basis for discussions. The motivation to change must come from the individual and not the healthcare professional in order for change to be successful. Any resistance or ambivalence to change needs to be discussed and resolved and the health professional should use encouragement to increase the patient's level of confidence in their ability to change. Interventions should be targeted at changing the attitude an individual has towards a behaviour rather than the behaviour itself. Part of the process involves getting the patient to set short-, medium-, and long-term goals and also looking at difficulties that might undermine behaviour change.

[19] Prochaska JO, DiClemente C (eds) (1984) *The Transtheoretical Approach: Crossing Traditional Foundations of Change*. Irwin, Homewood, IL.

[20] Miller WR, Rollnick S (1991) *Motivational Interviewing: Preparing People to Change Addictive Behavior*. Guilford Press, New York.

Concordance

Concordance is the term used to describe an agreement relating to treatment and lifestyle changes that is reached after negotiation and discussion between a patient and a healthcare professional. This approach signals a new relationship between patients and healthcare professionals and replaces the practice of viewing patients as either compliant or noncompliant. The compliance model relates to the extent to which patient behaviour coincides with health advice, but does not take into account the reasons for noncompliance. Examples of noncompliant behaviour include the failure to attend follow-up appointments, the failure to take medications correctly or renew prescriptions, and continuing harmful practices, such as smoking. Noncompliance can be total or partial; moreover, noncompliance might not be intentional. Nonintentional noncompliance might relate to the abilities of the patient—e.g. a patient might not recall or understand the health advice given. The patient might also lack the personal resources or motivation to change their behaviour or it might clash with their cultural or religious beliefs. The compliance model implies that healthcare professionals have authority over patients, that their views and advice are 'correct', and that patients' beliefs or wishes do not need to be considered.

It has long been recognized that rates of compliance (or noncompliance) vary widely, but it is generally agreed that compliance rates ↓ with time. The concordance model, however, places great emphasis on developing therapeutic alliances between patients and healthcare professionals, so that relationships are built up and maintained over time. The aim of concordance is to optimize health gain by the best use of medicines, therapies, or lifestyle changes compatible with what the patient desires or is capable of achieving.

In the concordance model, the healthcare professional is responsible for eliciting the patient's views and beliefs about their condition and their wishes relating to its future management. The healthcare professional needs to assess the patient's level of understanding about their condition, the personal resources available to them (physical, psychological, social, and financial), and their willingness and ability to make decisions about their care. The healthcare professional's role is obligatory and they are required to offer options based on the best available evidence. By contrast, the patient's role is voluntary, but they have a responsibility to honestly relate their views and to take responsibility for the consequences of their decisions.

The implementation of the concordance model relies on five goals:

- Healthcare professionals must view prescribing or planning as a joint venture with their patients.
- Patients should expect to be involved in decisions about their treatments.
- Resources should be available to help patients with different needs to understand the options available to them.
- Healthcare professionals should work in a collaborative manner with their patients and other healthcare and social care professionals.
- Services should be available to support patients in their endeavours relating to the management of their condition.

In moving towards the concordance model, healthcare professionals need to be mindful of allocating sufficient time to regular follow-up consultations, because the patient's views and abilities could change over time. The price of compliance was dependency. The price of concordance is the greater responsibility of the healthcare professional for the quality of consultations and of the patient for the consequences of their actions and decisions.

Related guidance

British Association for Cardiovascular Prevention and Rehabilitation (2012) *The BACPR Standards and Core Components for Cardiovascular Disease Prevention and Rehabilitation 2012* (2nd edn). BACPR, London.

British Heart Foundation (2011) *Trends in Coronary Heart Disease 1961 – 2011.* British Heart Foundation, London.

Department of Health (2008) *Putting Prevention First – Vascular Checks: Risk Assessment and Management.* DH, London.

Department of Health (2010) *Equity and Excellence: Liberating the NHS.* DH, London.

Department of Health (2013) *Cardiovascular Disease Outcome Strategy – improving outcomes for people with or at risk of cardiovascular disease.* DH, London.

Lai DT, Cahill K, Qin Y, Tang JL (2010) Motivational interviewing for smoking cessation. *Cochrane Database Systematic Review* 1, CD006936.

National Institute for Health and Clinical Excellence (2009) *Type 2 Diabetes: The Management of Type 2 Diabetes.* NICE, London.

National Institute for Health and Clinical Excellence (2010) *Prevention of Cardiovascular Disease – A National Framework for Action.* NICE, London

National Institute for Health and Clinical Excellence (2010) *Prevention of Cardiovascular Disease at Population Level.* NICE, London.

National Institute for Health and Clinical Excellence (2011) *Hypertension: Clinical Management of Primary Hypertension in Adults.* NICE, London.

Perk J, DeBacker G, Gohlke H, et al. for the Fifth Joint Task Force of the European Society of Cardiology and Other Societies on Cardiovascular Disease Prevention in Clinical Practice (2012) European Guidelines on cardiovascular disease prevention in clinical practice (version 2012). *European Heart Journal* 33, 1635–701.

Reiner Z, Catapano A, DeBacker G, et al. (2011) ESC/EAS guidelines for the management of dyslipidaemias. The Task Force on the management of dyslipidaemias of the European Society of Cardiology (ESC) and the European Atherosclerosis Society (EAS). *European Heart Journal* 32, 1769–818.

Scottish Intercollegiate Guideline Network (2010) *Management of Obesity: A National Clinical Guideline.* SIGN, Edinburgh.

Cardiac assessment

Introduction

It is essential that the cardiac nurse can carry out a comprehensive cardiac assessment of their patient. The nursing assessment aims to describe the patient's condition and help determine an accurate diagnosis, so that an effective and timely clinical management plan is implemented. The focus of the initial assessment varies according to the setting and clinical presentation of the patient. However, the priority is always to determine whether the patient is haemodynamically stable, whether they are suffering from an acute cardiac event that would benefit from time-dependent therapy, and the need for symptom management.

A thorough cardiac assessment requires the nurse to use a wide range of interpersonal, observational, and technical skills. Additionally, the nurse needs an in-depth knowledge of cardiac anatomy, physiology, and pathophysiology to determine the significance of the findings. The following elements should be included in the assessment:

- Observation of the patient
- Questioning to ascertain symptoms and immediate concerns of the patient
- Physical assessment (📖 Heart sounds, p.47; 📖 Breath sounds, p.59). This is usually performed by specialist nurses only
- History-taking, including relevant past medical history, medication history, social history, and assessment of cardiovascular risk factors (📖 Risk factors for cardiovascular disease, p.9)
- Diagnostic tests, which could indicate signs of heart disease, such as electrocardiogram (ECG) and blood tests.

This chapter outlines how to assess key symptoms and signs of cardiac disease. Symptoms are things that the patient reports as troublesome issues; signs are associated physiological changes that the health professional might discover during the course of their assessment.

General assessment of the patient

Always undertake a general assessment of the patient; however, the timing of the assessment depends on the healthcare setting and the severity of the patient's presenting symptoms. There are a variety of methods of assessment; it is unimportant which of these methods are used as long as the assessment is thorough and systematic (Ω Assessment of the deteriorating patient, p.335 for ABCDE method). A general assessment should include these points:

- Respiratory assessment (Ω Respiratory assessment p.57). What is the patient's breathing like? Are they dyspnoeic (Ω Dyspnoea, p.32)? Is cyanosis present?
- Observation of vital signs: BP (Ω Assessment of arterial blood pressure, p.35), HR (Ω Assessment of heart rate and arterial pulses, p.39), capillary refill time (CRT), 12-lead ECG (Ω 12-lead electrocardiogram (ECG), p.43).
- Level of response/consciousness/orientation.
- Are the neck veins distended? To assess this, the patient needs to be placed in a supine position and the head of the bead is then raised to 45°. Instruct the patient to turn their head away from you. A light shone across the neck may help in the assessment. The measurement is up from the manubriosternal angle to the where the vein is seen to be filled with blood (normal is <3cm).
- Is oedema evident? The best method of assessment for the presence of oedema is to press the ball of the thumb or tip of the index finger on the skin for a few seconds. If oedema is present, an indentation from the thumb or finger remains in the skin. This is called 'pitting oedema'. Oedema is most likely to be seen in the ankles, but can be present as high as the sacral area.
- Pain assessment (Ω Chest pain, p.28).
- Appearance and temperature of the skin—are signs of dehydration such as sunken eyes present? Does the skin feel cool, warm, or clammy?
- Body temperature measurement.
- Does the patient have xanthelasma (small, raised, yellowish plaques on and around the skin of the eyelids) or corneal arcus (a white ring surrounding the cornea), which are suggestive of hyperlipidaemia, or diagonal ear creases, which are suggestive of CHD?
- Nail and hand assessment—look for splinter haemorrhages, Osler's nodes, Janeway lesions (Ω Signs and symptoms, p.103) and clubbing of the nails (loss of nail-bed angle, ↑ curvature of nail and bulbous ends of fingers).
- Urinary output and urinalysis.
- Blood glucose level, if appropriate.
- BMI: BMI = weight (kg)/height^2 (m).
- Allergies.

Following the general assessment, the in-depth assessment of symptoms, physical examination, and further investigations can be commenced.

Chest pain

Chest pain is one of the cardinal symptoms of CHD, although not every patient with CHD presents with chest pain. For example, some patients with diabetes mellitus and elderly patients do not experience chest pain because of altered sensory perception. Angina is an ischaemic pain, which is caused by ↓ blood supply to the myocardium because of stenosed (narrowed) coronary arteries. It can, in some instances, result from aortic stenosis (AS), which causes inadequate perfusion of the coronary arteries, or from hypertrophic cardiomyopathy, whereby the myocardium has ↑ O_2 demands because of the ↑ in muscle mass.

The difficulty when patients report chest pain is in ascertaining whether the pain is cardiac in origin, because there are several other causes (📖 Differential diagnosis of chest pain, p.30). However, because some causes, such as MI and dissecting aortic aneurysm, can be life threatening, it is crucial that a differential diagnosis is made as quickly as possible so that appropriate treatments can be instigated. A 12-lead ECG must be recorded and reviewed for abnormalities such as ischaemia or infarction (📖 Analysing an ECG, p.45; 📖 Specific principles for nursing patients with ST-segment elevation ACS, p.126; and 📖 Specific principles for nursing patients with non-ST-segment elevation ACS, p.131). A systematic assessment of chest pain is required in patients presenting with chest pain. The 'PQRST' mnemonic is often used in assessment:

- P: precipitating, aggravating, and relieving factors—anginal pain is commonly associated with exertion, emotional distress, eating a heavy meal, or cold weather. It is, ∴, important to find out what the patient was doing when their chest pain started. It is also useful to ask if anything makes the pain worse. Asking what makes the pain disappear is also constructive—stable angina is usually relieved by glyceryl trinitrate (GTN) or rest. Angina at rest is indicative of acute coronary syndromes (ACS), especially if it is not relieved by GTN.
- Q: quality of pain—typically, anginal pain is described as crushing, constricting, vice-like, band-like, a tightness around the chest, or chest heaviness. Some patients do not experience pain, but describe either numbness or tingling, especially in the left arm. They might describe chest discomfort rather than pain. Some patients state that angina is like indigestion or heartburn. For these reasons, it is best to ask the patient to describe their symptoms rather than asking if they have pain. Associated symptoms—ask the patient if they have any other symptoms associated with the chest pain, such as breathlessness, dizziness, and sweating. The nurse should also observe for these and other related signs, such as pallor or tachycardia.
- R: region/radiation—angina is usually retrosternal, commonly radiating down the left arm and up into the neck. In some patients, pain might radiate to both arms, the jaw, shoulders, or the back.

- S: severity or intensity—although this is a subjective measure, it can help evaluate the efficacy of treatments or provide a comparison with previous episodes of pain. Various pain-assessment tools are available, but a commonly used tool is the numerical rating scale, whereby the patient is asked how severe their pain is on a scale of 0–10, with 0 being 'no pain' and 10 being 'the worst pain imaginable'. Some patients, however, can find it hard to give their pain a numerical value.
  ► Remember that there is not always a correlation between the severity of pain and the seriousness of the underlying disease.
  A patient with advanced triple-vessel disease could present with less pain than another patient who has a small single lesion.
- T: timing—► ascertain the length of time the patient has had the current bout of chest pain. Is the pain new in onset or have they experienced this type of pain before? The nurse should also ask if the discomfort began suddenly or whether the patient gradually became increasingly aware of it. If the patient has previously experienced chest pain, ask the patient how often they get the pain and whether there has been any change in its frequency, which might suggest progression of CHD.

Differential diagnosis of chest pain

Chest pain is the commonest reason for emergency calls and one of the most common reasons for seeking medical advice. It is important to recognize that there are causes of chest pain other than CHD. The differential diagnosis of chest pain relies on an assessment of both the chest pain itself, other associated signs and symptoms, and taking a thorough patient history (Table 2.1).

Table 2.1 Differential diagnosis of chest pain

Differential diagnosis	Symptoms and signs	Other information
Dissecting aortic aneurysm (📖 Aortic dissection, p.357)	Pain usually described as a 'tearing' or 'ripping' pain, which may radiate to the shoulder blades or back Peripheral pulses are often absent as the dissection progresses	Pain usually noted as sudden in onset
Pericarditis (📖 Acute pericarditis, p.310)	Pain is usually sharp Pain is worse when lying down and on inspiration Usually associated with pyrexia A pericardial rub might be heard	Pain is relieved by anti-inflammatory medication, e.g. non-steroidal anti-inflammatory drug (NSAID)
Pulmonary embolism (PE) (📖 Pulmonary embolism, p.344)	Pain occurs in relation to pulmonary infarction. It is associated with breathlessness and often collapse if a large PE has occurred	Assessment for risk factors for DVT should be considered, e.g. recent surgery or long haul flight
Pneumothorax (📖 Tension pneumothorax, p.346)	Usually, breathlessness is related to the size and type of the pneumothorax Pain is usually sharp and on affected side ↓ air entry on affected side Associated with breathlessness, pallor, and tachycardia	Risk factors for pneumothorax include chronic obstructive pulmonary disease (COPD), trauma, and tall, thin, young people
Pleuritic pain	Pain is usually stabbing or sharp and ↑ with coughing A pleural rub might be heard Often associated with pyrexia	May be related to recent pneumonia, PE or pneumothorax

Table 2.1 (Continued)

Differential diagnosis	Symptoms and signs	Other information
Sternal costochondritis	Chest tenderness over the affected joint, which worsens with pressure	May be the result of repeated minor trauma
Oesophageal reflux/oesophagitis	Usually described as a burning pain	Can be relieved by antacids
Gastric or duodenal ulceration	Usually epigastric pain associated with food intake	Often associated with weight loss
Anxiety	Stabbing pain associated with hyperventilation and sweating	Assessment of potential stressors important

Dyspnoea

Dyspnoea, or difficulty with breathing, is a common symptom of heart disease, in addition to respiratory disease (Table 2.2). It can also be caused by anaemia or malignant disease. Dyspnoea related to cardiac disease is usually associated with heart failure, which can be transient or chronic. It is related to the ↑ workload of breathing and overworked respiratory muscles. Pulmonary congestion reduces O_2 transfer and makes the lungs less compliant, which requires ↑ effort from respiratory muscles. Patients might describe dyspnoea variously as difficulty with breathing, breathlessness, or shortness of breath.

Note whether the patient is dyspnoeic at rest or on exertion. Patients might also report the following conditions:
• Orthopnoea—difficulty in breathing when lying flat.
• Paroxysmal nocturnal dyspnoea—the patient is awoken with breathlessness if they slide down the bed.

Pulmonary venous congestion causes both of these conditions, which are relieved if the patient sits upright. Prevent these conditions by ensuring several pillows support the patient.

If a patient presents with dyspnoea, undertake a full respiratory assessment (⩗ Respiratory assessment, p.57).

Table 2.2 Major causes of dyspnoea

Respiratory	COPD, asthma, pneumonia, pneumothorax, PE, lung cancer, and trauma
Cardiac	Acute left ventricular failure (LVF) and CHF
Neuromuscular	Muscular dystrophy and Guillain–Barré syndrome
Central nervous system	↑ intracranial pressure (ICP)
Endocrine	Diabetic ketoacidosis (DKA)-induced hyperventilation
Miscellaneous	Anaemia and obesity

Note that many patients might have dyspnoea caused by multiple pathologies, e.g. COPD and LVF.

Palpitations

Palpitations occur when the patient is aware of their own heartbeat and are described as a thumping in the chest, a racing heart, or an awareness of extra or irregular beats. ▶ Palpitations are not necessarily an indication of heart disease and it is, ∴, important to ascertain if they are associated with other symptoms, such as chest pain or breathlessness. Also determine if they occur at rest or on exertion, or if they are associated with other events, such as intake of caffeine, drugs, or alcohol. Of note, palpitations are not necessarily an indication of arrhythmia and patients with arrhythmias do not necessarily experience palpitations. ▶ Stress and anxiety are also often associated with palpitations because of catecholamine release and so it is important to determine if any stressors were present before the palpitations occurred.

If a patient presents with recurrent palpitations, it is usual to record a 12-lead ECG, preferably while the palpitations occur. Ambulatory electrocardiography (AECG) monitoring might be required to detect any associated arrhythmia (◻ Ambulatory monitoring, p.72).

In the acute setting continuous cardiac monitoring can facilitate the identification of arrhythmias. Telemetry may be used, if available. The patient's BP should also be recorded to detect any associated changes in cardiac output (CO). Palpation of the pulse also gives an indication of amplitude or volume.

Syncope

Syncope is a transient loss of consciousness (TLoC) caused by inadequate cerebral blood flow. Syncope presents in various forms:

- Neural mediated syncope (reflex syncope): TLoC due to a reflex bradycardic or hypotensive response. This includes vasovagal syncope, carotid sinus syncope, and situational syncope.
- Vasovagal or vasomotor syncope: caused by a combination of ↓ heart rate (HR) and vasodilatation, which results in ↓ CO and cerebral perfusion. It often occurs after prolonged standing, but can be associated with pain, retching, or emotion, and usually has warning signs of weakness, sweating, and nausea. Some patients experience a 'sinking feeling' before a syncopal attack, which is usually self-limiting because the person 'faints' and falls down, a posture that produces an improved cerebral blood flow. Frequent vasovagal syncope can be investigated using a 'tilt' test and a permanent pacemaker may be advised.
- Carotid sinus syncope: results from stimulation of the carotid sinus, which produces gross cardiac slowing and ↓ CO. This condition can occur because of restrictive clothing around the neck, especially in the elderly.
- Situational syncope occurs with certain situations. An example of this is micturition syncope. This occurs in older men, whereby syncope occurs after passing urine, usually at night. It is sometimes associated with ↑ alcohol consumption and is probably the result of ↓ venous return during straining to micturate and reflex vasodilatation 2° to the relief of an overdistended bladder.
- Arrhythmia-related syncope: a significant ↓ in CO after the onset of very fast or slow arrhythmias produces syncope. A particularly notable form of syncope is a Stokes–Adams attack associated with complete heart block. Brief periods of sinus arrest are superimposed on the heart block, which typically last ~15s.
- Convulsive syncope: transient inadequate cerebral flow accompanied by convulsive movements (usually the limbs).
- Syncope on exertion: usually associated with AS, whereby the narrowed valve seriously compromises CO at a time when O_2 demands are ↑. Can also be a feature of hypertrophic cardiomyopathy.
- Postural orthostatic tachycardia syndrome (PoTS): this is a disease of orthostatic intolerance. Sufferers will have symptoms such as dizziness, headaches, palpitations, that are relieved when lying down. It may present with recurrent syncopal episodes.

▶ As for patients presenting with other potential cardiac symptoms, it is important to ascertain the nature, frequency, and duration of any syncopal attacks. It is crucial to establish what activities occurred before the syncopal episodes and identify any associated symptoms. Any episodes of confusion or convulsions must also be noted. Record BP, HR, and 12-lead ECG. NICE have produced guidelines[1] on the assessment, diagnosis and management of TLoC.

---

[1] National Institute for Health and Clinical Excellence (2010) *Transient Loss of Consciousness*. NICE, London. ℘ http://www.nice.org.uk

Assessment of arterial blood pressure

BP is the force exerted by the blood on the walls of arteries in which it is contained. The elasticity and width of the blood vessels and the ability of the heart to expel the blood govern BP. ∴, BP is related directly to CO and peripheral resistance. ► BP is one of the most commonly recorded clinical observations and is an important indicator of cardiac function. It is also a predictor of mortality and morbidity.

BP can be measured directly, by placing a cannula with a pressure transducer into an artery (☐ Arterial monitoring, p.37) or indirectly, by using aneroid or electronic sphygmomanometers. Arterial BP monitoring provides the most accurate measurement, but it is invasive and thus not practicable in most clinical situations. Reserve this method of BP monitoring for patients with critical care needs.

A sphygmomanometer is the most commonly used method of measuring BP in clinical practice. Measuring BP manually is relatively straightforward, however, there are several potential sources of inaccuracy or bias, but these can be reduced (Table 2.3).

Numerous factors influence BP, greatly depending on the characteristics of the individual patient (e.g. age and weight).

- The normal range for adult BP is as follows:
  - Systolic: 90–140mmHg.
  - Diastolic: 60–90mmHg.
- Hypotension (low BP): can lead to inadequate perfusion of the vital organs and tissues. Causes include haemorrhage, cardiogenic shock, LVF, sepsis, and drugs (e.g. opiates and nitrates).
- Hypertension (high BP): ↑ the workload of the myocardium. Causes include obesity and renal disease.

❶ Consider that due to physiological changes the older adult patient may actually be hypotensive with a 'normal' BP.

► In both hypotension and hypertension, it is important to assess other vital signs to determine the probable cause of the abnormality, because the body has compensatory mechanisms. For example, a ↓ in circulating blood volume initially results in an ↑ in HR to maintain BP.

Table 2.3 Potential sources of error in manual BP monitoring

Source	Potential error	Factors reducing error
Nurse	• Poor sight or hearing • Poor understanding of the procedure	• Sphygmomanometer at eye level • Stethoscope not touching cuff during procedure • Good education and supervision
Patient	• Diurnal variation • Restrictive clothing • 'White coat syndrome'	• Regular recording of BP • No tight clothing on arm • Rested and calm
Equipment	• Incorrect size of cuff • Faulty valves • Lack of calibration	• Cuff bladder of correct size to cover at least 80% of the arm's circumference • Sphygmomanometer regularly maintained and calibrated
Technique	• Lack of arm support • Incorrect cuff application • Poor valve control	• Arm supported at heart level • Centre of bladder in cuff placed over brachial artery • Lower edge of cuff 2–3cm above antecubital fossa • Good education and supervision

Electronic sphygmomanometers must be regularly calibrated and maintained.

Arterial monitoring

Arterial monitoring records BP more accurately. It gives a constant recording of systolic BP, diastolic BP, and mean arterial pressure (MAP).

$$MAP = \frac{systolic\ BP\ +\ (2 \times diastolic\ BP)}{3}$$

Normal range: 70–105mgHg.

Use arterial monitoring in the following situations and patient groups:

- Critically ill patients
- Haemodynamically unstable patients
- Cardiac surgery
- Major surgery, e.g. abdominal or neurological surgery
- If the patient is receiving potent vasodilators, vasopressors or inotropes
- If regular arterial blood gases are required
- When the patient has an intra-aortic balloon pump (IABP) *in situ*
- Shock
- It should only be used where staff can interpret results.

Arterial monitoring is contraindicated in patients with haemorrhagic disorders.

Although the radial artery is the most common site for placement of the arterial line, the femoral, brachial, and dorsalis pedis arteries are also used. Before insertion in the radial artery, perform a modified Allan's test to ensure good arterial flow to the hand (occlude the radial artery to assess ulna flow).

Once the arterial cannula is in place, it needs constant flushing with saline. The bag of fluid should be placed in a pressure bag and the pressure kept at 300mmHg to deliver 3mL/hr. Zero the transducer at the phlebostatic axis and keep the same reference point each time the transducer is zeroed. A non-invasive BP measurement is usually also recorded once per shift.

A normal arterial tracing is shown in Fig. 2.1. Poor ventricular contraction, hypotension, occlusion or kinking of the line, loss of transducer pressure, or arrhythmias can dampen the waveform.

Complications of arterial lines include the following:

- Haemorrhage
- Infection
- Necrosis
- Vascular insufficiency
- Emboli or thrombus formation
- Cannula displacement
- Oedema
- Drug or fluid administration in the line.

Nursing care

- Observe the site for complications, as already described.
- Cover the site with a transparent occlusive dressing.
- Clean the site and change the dressing as required: a local protocol should be in place for associated line changes, swabbing for microscopy, sensitivity, & culture (M,C&S) and cannula re-insertion.
- Label the arterial line clearly.
- Check that all connections are secure.
- Keep the line continuously flushed using a pressure-bag system (500mL of normal saline at 300mmHg).
- Zero the system each time the patient changes position.
- Perform a 'square wave' test (fast flush and release of flush device and observation of the resulting 'square' waveform) to establish if there is an optimally damped trace and to troubleshoot accordingly. Overdamping will underestimate systolic pressure and underdamping will overestimate systolic pressure. Overdamped arterial waveforms typically have a blunted, slurred form and loss of dicrotic notch. Underdamped arterial waveforms have an overshoot spike which exaggerates the upstroke of the waveform and additional artefacts ('ringing').
- Observe peripheral perfusion.
- Always flush the line well following arterial blood sampling.
- Check that monitor alarms are set appropriately and are turned on.
- Check the patient and the equipment if the trace becomes flat.
- Where possible, the cannula should remain visible at all times and care taken when moving or turning the patient as it can easily become dislodged.

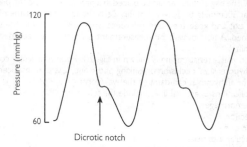

Fig. 2.1 Arterial trace. Reproduced from Chikwe J, Beddow E, and Glenville B. *Cardiothoracic Surgery*, OUP, 2006. By permission of Oxford University Press.

Assessment of heart rate and arterial pulses

The HR can be noted from a cardiac monitor; however, this does not give any qualitative information about the arterial pulse. A normal ECG trace may not be producing a cardiac output as in pulseless electrical activity (PEA) (📖 Resuscitation, p.339). ▶∴, palpate an arterial pulse. The radial pulse is the most common site for palpation because it is easily accessed. However, if the patient has a low CO, the radial pulse might be difficult to palpate, so use the carotid or femoral pulses instead. Palpate the pulse for a full 1min the first time it is assessed. If the pulse is regular, palpate for 30s and double the number. The frequency of pulse recording depends on the patient's condition; the pulse is most useful when noted in conjunction with the BP.

Note the following characteristics of the pulse:

Rate

The normal resting HR is usually between 60–80bpm, although an HR up to 100bpm is considered to be within the normal range. A rate <60bpm (bradycardia) is usually sinus bradycardia, which could either be due to heart block or be the result of drugs, such as β-blockers. Athletes often have a slow resting pulse. A rate >100bpm (tachycardia) is often associated with exertion or emotion. If the HR is >120bpm at rest, suspect an underlying problem (e.g. arrhythmia, haemorrhage). Heart transplant recipients are generally tachycardic at rest 90–120bpm due to the denervation of the transplanted heart.

Rhythm

The pulse should be regular. Variation of the pulse with inspiration and expiration is 'sinus arrhythmia' and is not of concern. If the pulse is irregular, note the pattern of the irregularity (i.e. is it irregularly irregular, whereby the next pulse cannot be anticipated, or is it regularly irregular, whereby the next pulse can be anticipated). An example of a regularly irregular pulse might be one where every fourth beat is missing.

Volume or amplitude

The amplitude of the pulse directly relates to the pulse pressure, i.e. the difference between the systolic BP and the diastolic BP. The pulse should be easily palpable. The following abnormalities might be noted:

- Low pulse volume—usually because of a ↓ CO or ↑ peripheral resistance.
- High pulse volume—usually because of high output states, such as anaemia, pregnancy, and hyperthyroidism.
- Waterhammer pulse—a collapsing pulse associated with AR.
- Pulsus biferiens—felt as a slow, rising-and-collapsing pulse. This is indicative of combined AR and AS.
- Pulsus alternans—strong and weak pulse waves that alternate in a regular rhythm. This is indicative of serious heart disease.

Indicators of cardiac output

The performance of the heart's pumping ability is described in terms of the CO, which is the volume of blood pumped by one ventricle in 1min. It is equivalent to the stroke volume (SV) multiplied by the number of contractions per minute (HR):

CO = SV × HR.

Normal CO is ~5L/min.

There are methods of directly measuring CO (⊞ Pulmonary artery pressure monitoring: 1, p.53), but there are other indirect measurements that help in the assessment of CO. An ↑ HR and ↓ urine output (<0.5mL/kg/h) are good indicators of a ↓ CO. BP gives some indication of CO. If CO ↓, BP will eventually ↓ as well. The capillary refill test (CRT) also gives an indication of CO and is a good indicator of fluid status and peripheral perfusion. Perform this test on the nail beds by applying pressure until blanching occurs. Then remove the pressure and measure the time taken for the nail bed to return to a pink colour. The colour should return in <2s. However, remember that a slow CRT might simply be an indication of PVD or vasoconstriction resulting from a low room temperature.

Cardiac monitoring

Cardiac monitoring provides continuous tracing of the patient's HR and rhythm. It is widely used both in the pre-hospital and hospital setting. However, do not use cardiac monitoring in isolation. Because cardiac monitoring normally only shows a single lead, perform a 12-lead ECG if ischaemia or infarction is suspected and to give a better picture of any rhythm abnormalities. Many cardiac monitors also monitor oxygen saturation (SaO_2), non-invasive BP, and respiration. More sophisticated monitors enable monitoring of arterial pressures, central venous pressure (CVP), CO studies and pulmonary artery pressures. Indications for cardiac monitoring include the following:

- Surgery—both during surgery and immediately postoperatively
- Chest pain
- Suspected ACS
- Critically ill patients
- Post-MI
- During and following cardiac arrest
- Rhythm abnormalities
- Poisoning and overdose.

Both three-lead and five-lead monitoring systems can be used. The principles of monitoring are the same for each system. To maintain good electrode contact, the patient's skin needs to be dry and excessive hair shaved. Change electrodes every 24–72h to prevent the gel from drying out and the patient's skin from becoming sore. Place electrodes over bone and not muscle, avoiding areas where defibrillation pads or paddles might be placed if required. All connections should be checked, in addition to the gain on the monitor, to ensure that the ECG complex can be seen. It is usual to monitor in lead II. Set the alarms on the monitor. Both shivering ('somatic tremor' = irregular baseline artefact) and electrical pumps (AC supply = thick baseline artefact) can cause interference.

If a three-lead system is used, place the red electrode at the right shoulder, with the yellow electrode to the left shoulder and the green electrode on the left-hand side of the abdomen. If a five-lead system is used, the first three leads are placed, as just outlined, and then the black lead is placed on the right-hand side of the abdomen and the white (respiratory) lead is placed in the middle of the patient's chest.

ST-segment monitoring

This is available on many cardiac monitors and measures ST-segment deviation from the isoelectric line. It is particularly useful in detecting silent ischaemia, effectiveness of reperfusion therapy, and recurrent ischaemia post MI. Use of ST-segment monitoring is variable.

Telemetry

Telemetry systems enable monitoring of the patient while they are mobile. Attach the telemetry system in the same way, as outlined earlier, but the patient carries the telemetry box with them. The rhythm can be observed on a monitor, either on the same ward or on a ward nearby. It is important to be aware of safety aspects of telemetry such as the fact that although the rhythm can be observed the patient may not always be seen, for example, if they are on a different ward. Change the batteries regularly.

Reading a rhythm strip

Use a systematic approach to analyse the rhythm strip which covers the following:

- Is there electrical activity? If not, check the patient, leads, electrodes, and gain on the monitor.
- Check the rate: each large square = 0.20s and each small square = 0.04s. To calculate the rate, count the number of QRS complexes within a 6s strip (30 large squares) and multiply this number by 10 (this will = HR).
- Check the regularity of the rhythm: place a sheet of plain paper over a rhythm strip, mark off three QRS complexes and move the paper along to match the marks to the next set of complexes. If the rhythm is irregular, look for patterns, e.g. is it irregularly or regularly irregular?
- Look for atrial activity: there should be one P-wave to each QRS complex. Check the morphology of the P-wave, which should be gently rounded. A wide, notched P-wave indicates left atrial hypertrophy (LAH) and a pointed P-wave indicates right atrial hypertrophy (RAH). If there is no atrial activity, look for a junctional rhythm (⎚ Sinus bradycardia and sino-atrial node disease, p.215). If there is a saw-tooth appearance, it is probably atrial flutter (⎚ Atrial flutter, p.249). Chaotic atrial activity usually indicates AF (⎚ Atrial fibrillation, p.247).
- Check the P–R interval: it should be 0.12–0.20s (3–5 small squares). If it is >0.20s, first-degree heart block is present (⎚ Atrioventricular blocks: first-degree heart block, p.217).
- Look at the QRS complex: it should be no wider than 0.11s. A widened QRS complex might result from left and/or right bundle branch block (⎚ Bundle branch block, p.221) or indicate a ventricular rhythm or aberrant conduction (⎚ SVT with aberrant conduction, p.251).
- Check if there is a T wave and if it looks normal. Examine the QT interval it should be <half preceding R–R interval. If the rhythm is very fast T waves may not be visible.

12-lead electrocardiogram (ECG)

The 12-lead ECG gives a more three-dimensional view of the heart compared to standard cardiac monitoring. It is usually a one-off recording, although use serial recordings in the event of an MI. ► Place the ECG electrodes in the same position each time to enable accurate recording and ECG comparison.

ECGs measure the change in current within the heart. If an electrode is placed on the surface of the heart and attached to an ECG machine, the trace will show an upwards deflection if the impulse is travelling towards it and downwards if the impulse travels away from it. This is because the heart muscle has different directions of force (or vectors). The largest electrical current flows from the base to the apex of the heart in a right to left direction.

Recording an ECG

The patient should be relaxed and remain still while the recording takes place. Remove excess hair and moisture from the patient's skin. Record the ECG and label it with the patient's name, hospital number (if appropriate), date and time, and any other relevant information, such as the presence of chest pain and BP.

Limb leads

There are four limb leads. Place the red lead on the right arm, the yellow lead on the left arm, the green lead on the left leg, and the black lead on the right leg. The electrodes placed on the limbs give rise to the unipolar and bipolar leads.

Unipolar leads

Unipolar leads record the electrical potential in one direction only, towards an exploring electrode. The exploring electrode is placed on one limb and the negative pole connects to the central terminal via the other two limbs to augment the voltage of the tracing.

Augmented (amplified) vector (direction) right (aVR)

aVR records changes in potential in the part of the heart facing the right shoulder.

Augmented vector left (aVL)

aVL records changes in potential in the part of the heart facing the left shoulder.

Augmented vector foot (aVF)

aVF records changes in potential in the part of the heart facing the left hip.

Bipolar leads

The bipolar leads are attached to the right and left arms and the left foot. The lead attached to the right foot is an earth lead. The bipolar leads measure the potential between two points: positive and negative poles.

Lead I

Lead I measures the difference in potential between right and left arms.

Lead II

Lead II measures the difference in potential between right arm and left leg.

Lead III

Lead III measures the difference in potential between left arm and left leg.

Einthoven's triangle

Einthoven regarded each limb used in recording the bipolar ECG as an apex of an equilateral triangle, equidistant electrically from the heart at the centre.

The actual position of the bipolar limb leads is the sum of the potentials between one lead and those that would be obtained from an electrode diametrically opposite the other lead. The resultant force is directed midway between the two points (Fig. 2.2).

Precordial or chest leads

These are unipolar leads. The exploring electrode is placed over the chest (Fig. 2.3) and the indifferent electrode is connected to the limbs.

- V1—fourth intercostal space at the right sternal border.
- V2—fourth intercostal space at the left sternal border.
- V3—midway between V2 and V4.
- V4—fifth intercostal space on the midclavicular line.
- V5—fifth intercostal space on the anterior axillary line.
- V6—fifth intercostal space on the midaxillary line.

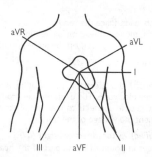

Fig. 2.2 Limb leads. Adapted with permission from Chikwe J, Beddow E, and Glenville B (2006). *Cardiothoracic Surgery*. Oxford University Press, Oxford.

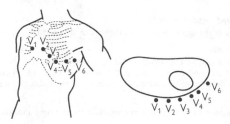

Fig. 2.3 Positions of the chest leads. Adapted with permission from Chikwe J, Beddow E, and Glenville B (2006). *Cardiothoracic Surgery*. Oxford University Press, Oxford.

Analysing an ECG

Fig. 2.4 shows a normal ECG. Use a systematic approach to analyse the ECG which covers the following:

- Check the standardization: the speed at 25mm/s. The voltage should be 10mm = 1mV (2 large squares).
- Check if there is a complete calibration pulse either at the beginning or end of each line this should indicate all lead sets are equally calibrated.
- Check patient ID against ECG.
- Analyse the rhythm strip (📖 Reading a rhythm strip, p.42).
- Lead aVR should be negative and lead II should be positive.
- Look at the axis:
  - Look at lead I and aVF.
  - If lead I is positive and aVF is positive = normal axis.
  - If lead I is positive and aVF is negative = left-axis deviation.
  - If lead I is negative and aVF is positive = right-axis deviation.
  See Table 2.4 for causes of right- and left-axis deviation.
- P-wave—normally <3mm tall and 3mm wide. It should be positive in the limb leads (not aVR) and V2–V6. It should also be gently rounded, not notched or pointed.
- P–R interval: 0.12–0.2s.
- The Q-wave should be <0.04s and <2mm deep.
- QRS complexes should be positive in leads I, II, and III and aVR. Large QRS complexes (tall R-waves and deep S-waves) could indicate hypertrophy.
- R-wave progression should ↑ from V2–V4. Poor R-wave progression might result from MI, LVH, and LBBB.
- The QRS complex should be <0.11s.
- ST segment: isoelectric, but might be slightly elevated (1mm) in V1 and V2. Elevation in other leads >1mm could indicate infarction (📖 Specific principles for nursing patients with ST-segment elevation ACS, p.126). Depression could indicate ischaemia (📖 Specific principles for nursing patients with non-ST-segment elevation ACS, p.131).
- The T-wave should be positive in leads with a positive QRS complex. It is normally positive in V3–V6 and lead II (depends on axis) and negative in aVR. It is usually no >5mm in limb leads and no >10mm in chest leads. It should also be slightly rounded, not pointed or notched.
- Measure the QT interval from the beginning of the Q-wave to the end of the T-wave. It varies with HR, age and gender, but should be < one-half of the preceding R–R interval. The normal interval length is 0.35–0.42s, which is prolonged by myocardial ischaemia, hypocalcaemia, and hypokalaemia and shortened by digitalis and hypercalcaemia.
- The U-wave is best seen in V3. Prominent U-waves are observed in hypokalaemia. Negative U-waves with positive T-waves strongly suggest left main stem (LMS) stenosis.

Table 2.4 Causes of right and left axis deviation

Left axis deviation	Right axis deviation
• Left anterior hemiblock	• Left posterior hemiblock
• Inferior MI	• RVH
• VT	• PE
• WPW	

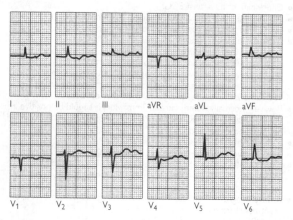

Fig. 2.4 Normal ECG. Reproduced with permission from Chikwe J, Beddow E, and Glenville B (2006). *Cardiothoracic Surgery.* Oxford University Press, Oxford.

Heart sounds

Examination of the heart includes inspection, palpation, and auscultation. Evaluation of heart sounds forms the latter part of this assessment. Auscultation is a skill that more nurses are performing, but unless practised regularly, it can be a difficult skill to master and maintain. It is essential to use a good-quality stethoscope with a bell to listen to low-pitched sounds and diaphragm to distinguish high-pitched sounds. The areas for auscultation are linked to where the sound is produced and any turbulent blood flow radiates. The stethoscope is therefore placed in each of the following locations (Fig. 2.5):

- Second intercostal space, right sternal border—aortic area.
- Second intercostal space, left sternal border—pulmonary area.
- Fourth intercostal, space left sternal border—tricuspid area.
- Fifth intercostal space, left midclavicular line—mitral area.
- Third intercostal space, left sternal border—Erb's point (many heart murmurs will be heard better here).

Heart sounds are described as first (S_1), second (S_2), third (S_3), and fourth (S_4) sounds according to their position within systole and diastole. The time interval between S_2 and S_1 is longer than the interval between S_1 and S_2 because diastole is normally longer than systole. Palpate the carotid or radial pulse when auscultating—the heart sound heard when you first feel the pulse is S_1 and when it disappears, S_2. Each sound occurs as follows:

- S_1 marks the approximate beginning of ventricular systole, with the sudden closure of the tricuspid and mitral valves. These sounds are normally heard together; however, it is useful to remember that the MV closes just before the tricuspid valve. Listen at the apex to hear this sound more clearly.
- S_2 signifies the end of ventricular systole, with closure of the aortic valve and pulmonary valve. As just described, these sounds are normally heard together but, in fact, the aortic valve closes just before the pulmonary valve. This is usually prominent on deep inspiration, which causes a physiological splitting of the sound (↑ thoracic pressure and ↑ venous return). Listen at the left sternal edge with the diaphragm to hear this better—'lub d/dub' on inspiration.
- S_3 is heard during diastole and is linked to ventricular filling. It is a thumping, low-pitched sound and can be physiological (e.g. with pyrexia and in pregnancy) or pathological (e.g. left ventricular failure or aortic regurgitation). In cardiac failure, there is often associated tachycardia, which causes S_1 and S_2 to be quieter, and the rhythm is described as a 'gallop rhythm'—'lub-dub-dum'
- S_4 is a soft, low pitched sound that precedes S_1 and corresponds with atrial contraction. It is less common and always pathological. It may be heard in patients with aortic stenosis, hypertension and left ventricular hypertrophy—'da-lub-dub'

Heart sounds can be loud (e.g. S_1 in pyrexia) or soft (e.g. S_1 in tachycardia) or of variable intensity (e.g. S_1 in AF and complete heart block).

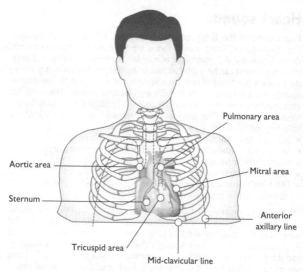

Fig. 2.5 Locations for auscultating heart sounds. Adapted with permission from Spiers C (2011) Cardiac auscultation. *British Journal of Cardiac Nursing* 6(10), 482–6. © MA Healthcare.

Extra heart sounds

These are described as 'clicks', 'snaps', murmurs, and rubs. They may occur as follows:

- An ejection click indicates stenosis of either aortic or pulmonary valves and is heard after S_1 as the malformed valve suddenly opens.
- A click midsystole (between S_1 and S_2) occurs with a prolapse, usually of the MV where the long chordae tendineae are no longer effective.
- An 'opening snap' is caused by a stenosed MV as it suddenly stops opening normally. It is, ∴, early diastolic in origin and heard following S_2.

Murmurs

Murmurs are heard during systole or diastole caused by turbulent flow across an abnormal valve, septal defect, or outflow obstruction or ↑ stroke volume through a normal valve. Murmurs may occur in a healthy heart and are termed 'innocent' (athletes, pregnancy, pyrexia).

It is important to note the timing (systolic or diastolic), duration (e.g. pansystolic), character and pitch (e.g. harsh, rumbling, high/low pitch), intensity (see bullet list), location (site heard best), and if there is any specific radiation (see bullet list) across the precordium. Also note any change of intensity during respiration—right heart murmurs are emphasized on inspiration.

- Grades of murmur intensity (Levine scale):
  - Grade 1—low intensity and difficult to hear, even by experts.
  - Grade 2—low intensity, but audible with a stethoscope (no palpable thrill).
  - Grade 3—medium intensity and easily heard with a stethoscope.
  - Grade 4—loud and audible (palpable thrill).
  - Grade 5—very loud but cannot be heard outside the precordium (palpable thrill).
  - Grade 6—audible with the stethoscope away from the chest.
- Radiation of sound follows the direction of the blood flow causing the murmur:
  - AS radiates to the aortic area and carotid arteries.
  - Mitral regurgitation radiates towards the left axilla.
  - VSD radiates towards the right sternal edge.
- Systolic murmurs:
  - A systolic murmur occurs if there is insufficiency of the MV or tricuspid valve or a VSD.
  - Aortic stenosis.
  - Increase in flow, e.g. pregnancy.
  - Murmurs are termed pansystolic (mitral or tricuspid regurgitation, VSD), midsystolic, or late systolic (MV prolapse).
  - An ejection systolic murmur is associated with ↑ blood flow through a normal aortic or pulmonary valve or normal flow through valves that are stenosed. This murmur quietly rises, crescendos mid-systole, and fades.

- Diastolic murmurs:
  - An early diastolic murmur has a decrescendo sound quality usually caused by aortic regurgitation (AR), (e.g. in Marfan's syndrome, syphilis, rheumatic heart disease, IE). It has a blowing, decrescendo quality best heard if the patient sits forward and breathes out fully, with the bell of the stethoscope at the lower left sternal border. Pulmonary regurgitation is rare (pulmonary hypertension or congenital defect).
  - A mid-diastolic murmur has a low pitched, rumbling sound that can be associated with an opening snap and is usually caused by mitral stenosis. It is best heard by placing the bell of the stethoscope at the apex of the heart while the patient is lying on their left side.
  - An Austin Flint murmur is a mid-diastolic murmur linked to aortic regurgitation. It is caused by regurgitant flow striking the MV and restricting inflow to the LV.
- Innocent (systolic) murmurs are not linked to an abnormality. They are common in children and young adults and are always quiet. Other cardiac findings (e.g. ECG and chest X-ray [CXR]) are normal.

Pericardial rub

The heart beating against an inflamed pericardium, e.g. in Dressler's syndrome (🕮 Acute pericarditis, p.310), causes a pericardial rub. The sound is continuous and heard across the precordium. It is usually louder when the patient leans forward. If the rub disappears when the patient holds their breath, it is more likely to be pleural in origin.

Prosthetic valves

Depending on the position, e.g. MV or aortic valve and type of valve (e.g. ball and cage or tilting disc), the artificial heart valve is heard distinctly as it opens and closes during systole and diastole. The closing sound is louder, described as metallic, and high pitched. Sounds may be palpable and audible without a stethoscope.

Central venous lines

Central venous lines can be used to record the CVP and for the administration of intravenous (IV) drugs and fluids. The CVP indicates the filling pressure of the right atrium and, hence, the preload. Record the CVP either continuously, using a transducer, or intermittently, using a manometer line. The central line is usually placed in either the internal jugular vein or subclavian vein; there is an ↑ risk of infection and greater discomfort for the patient if the femoral vein is used. However the femoral site may be used in an emergency situation such as cardiac arrest or when there is no other central access available. CVP lines can be single lumen or multi lumen. CVP lines are used for the following reasons:

- Administration of some IV drugs, e.g. amiodarone, inotropes
- Parenteral feeding
- CVP measurement
- Rapid fluid resuscitation
- Poor peripheral venous access
- Transvenous pacing access.

In health, the normal CVP is as follows:
- Transduced: 2–6mmHg (mid axilla) 0–8mmHg (right atrial level)
- Manometer: 5–10cmH$_2$O (midaxilla).

CVP is ↑ by the following factors:
- Fluid overload
- Right heart failure
- PE
- Pulmonary oedema
- Pulmonary hypertension
- Cardiac tamponade
- LVF.

CVP is ↓ by the following factors:
- Hypovolaemia
- Drug-induced venodilatation
- Sepsis
- Haemorrhage.

Whether using a transducer or manometer system, take recordings with the patient in the same position (supine if possible) and use the same reference point (to zero), usually midaxilla (can be the sternal angle). This will ensure that readings are consistent and comparable. Turn off all infusions or use a separate lumen to ensure accurate recordings and to prevent inadvertent bolus administration of drugs.

If using a manometer system, the procedure is as follows:
- Wash and dry hands.
- The line should be flushed to ensure it is patent.
- Position the patient supine.
- Ensure the arm of the manometer is level with the midaxilla. The bubble in the spirit level should be between the two lines.

- Switch the three-way tap 'on' to the manometer and fluid bag and 'off' to the patient.
- Fill the manometer tube slowly with fluid, until the level is just above the ~CVP.
- Turn the three-way tap 'on' to the patient and manometer and 'off' to the fluid, so that the fluid level falls in the manometer tube.
- Read the measurement when the fluid level has stopped falling. The fluid level may rise and fall slightly with respirations.
- When CVP has been recorded, turn the three-way tap back to the original position.

Nursing care

- Label lines clearly.
- 'Zero' line after patient has moved position (transduced) and before taking a reading (manometer).
- Observe the site for signs of bleeding, catheter displacement, infection, and swelling.
- Use a clean non-touch technique and gloves when handling the line.
- Clean the site using 2% chlorhexidine gluconate (check line manufacturer's exceptions).
- Change transparent dressing using an aseptic technique 24h post insertion and then every 7 days (sooner if moisture is underneath or not intact)—gauze dressings should be assessed daily and changed to transparent as soon as possible.
- Keep the catheter flushed. Aspirate to check blood return on the line before flushing and to assess patency. If a continuous infusion is not running, flush the line every 8–12h.
- Flush the line after given IV drug boluses and ensure the line is cleared when continuous infusions are complete, to prevent accidental bolus—withdraw 5–10mL, discard aspirate and then flush.
- Observe all connections are intact.
- Monitor the patient for complications, such as infection, pneumothorax, air embolism, haematoma, arrhythmias, and extravasation.
- When removing the line, the patient should be supine. The nurse should be wearing gloves and may need to clean the site after removing the sterile dressing (check local policy). Ask the patient to take a deep breath and hold it (to prevent an air embolism). Remove the catheter while applying pressure with some sterile gauze. The catheter should be inspected for any clots, breakages or signs of infection. Cover the site with a sterile, occlusive dressing. If an infection is present or suspected, send the tip of the line for culture and sensitivity.

Pulmonary artery pressure monitoring: 1

A pulmonary artery (PA) catheter is used to measure the pressure on the right side of the heart. When the tip of the catheter is wedged in a branch of the PA, it indicates the pressure on the left side of the heart (pulmonary artery wedge pressure (PAWP)). The catheter can also be used to facilitate calculation of CO.

The following are indications for PA catheters:
• Cardiogenic shock
• Complicated cardiac surgery
• Right ventricular failure (RVF)
• Pulmonary oedema (that fails to respond to therapy)
• Sepsis
• Major trauma
• Assessment of circulating volume
• CO studies
• Mixed venous O_2 saturation recording.

Contraindications for PA catheters include the following:
• Risks of PA catheter outweigh benefits
• Severe coagulation disorders
• A prosthetic right-heart valve
• An endocardial pacemaker (new)
• If staff cannot interpret results.

The catheter is usually inserted into either the right subclavian vein or the internal jugular vein. As the catheter passes through the right side of the heart, the waveform changes (Fig. 2.6). The normal values are as follows:
• RA pressure 0–8mmHg.
• RV systolic pressure 15–25mmHg and diastolic pressure 0–8mmHg (usually only seen during catheter insertion).
• PA systolic pressure 15–25mmHg and diastolic pressure 6–12mmHg:
  • Causes of ↑ PA pressure include LVF, pulmonary hypertension, fluid overload and some congenital heart diseases.
  • Hypovolaemia causes ↓ PA pressure.
• PAWP 4–12mmHg:
  • Causes of ↑ PAWP include fluid overload, LVF, and MV problems.
  • Hypovolaemia causes ↓ PAWP.

Once the catheter is inserted, a CXR is recorded to detect if complications, such as pneumothorax, have occurred. Keep the line continuously flushed using a pressure-bag system (500mL of normal saline at 300mmHg). Zero the system each time the patient changes position.

Cardiac output studies

CO can be recorded using thermodilution: cold fluid is injected quickly into the RA through the proximal port, and changes in temperature occur as the fluid passes through the heart. Perform the study three times and record the average.

Alternate methods of measuring cardiac output include pulse contour cardiac output[2] (PiCCO), lithium indicator dilution cardiac output[3] (LiDCO) and CardioQ-ODM[4] oesophageal Doppler monitor. CeVOX,[5] measures continuous venous O_2 saturations, which is especially useful in septic patients.

Nursing care

Observe the tracing regularly to ensure that the catheter is not wedged accidentally, because this causes damage to the PA. The site is a source of infection; ∴, clean the site using 2% chlorhexidine gluconate and change the dressing as required, most PA catheters are removed after 72h. If sheaths are left *in situ* cover with a transparent dressing and treat as a central line (🕮 Central venous lines, p.51). Observe the site for bleeding, swelling, redness, and signs of infection. Take care not to disconnect the lines and clearly label all lines to prevent mixing of infusions. Also observe for the following complications:

- Pneumothorax—which might occur on insertion
- Air embolism
- Thrombus formation
- Arrhythmias
- Heart block
- Balloon rupture
- Formation of vegetation
- Sepsis.

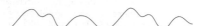

Fig. 2.6 CVP trace. Adapted with permission from Chikwe J, Beddow E, and Glenville B (2006). *Cardiothoracic Surgery*. Oxford University Press, Oxford.

---

[2] ⌕ http://www.healthcare.philips.com/gb_en/products/patient_monitoring/products/picco (accessed 31 October 2012)

[3] ⌕ http://www.lidco.com/clinical/lidco_science/lithium_dilution.php (accessed 31 October 2012).

[4] National Institute for Health and Clinical Excellence (2011) *CardioQ-ODM Oesophageal Doppler Monitor.* NICE, London. ⌕ http://www.nice.org.uk

[5] ⌕ http://www.pulsion.com/index.php?id=2648 (accessed 31 October 2012).

Pulmonary artery pressure monitoring 2: pulmonary artery wedge pressure

PAWP recording

The PAWP should reflect left ventricular end-diastolic pressure (LVEDP), unless the patient has pulmonary venous obstruction or MS. Use the following procedure to wedge the balloon:

- Using the attached syringe, inflate the balloon slowly according to the manufacturer's guidelines (usually not >1.5mL air).
- Observe the monitor for a change in the waveform (Fig. 2.7).
- With the balloon inflated, allow the trace to run for no more than 15s. A sharp rise in the trace indicates the balloon is overwedged.
- Freeze the monitor then deflate the balloon. Align the monitor cursor to the end of expiration on the waveform.
- Read and document the results.
- Unfreeze the monitor.
- Check the PA waveform has returned.

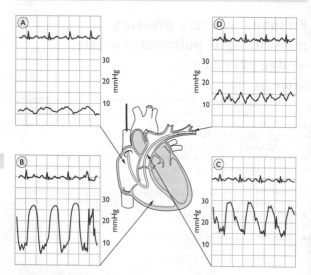

Right heart catheterization. In each panel, the ECG is shown at the top with the corresponding pressure trace from the distal port of a PA catheter at the bottom. The characteristic pressure traces indicate the position of the catheter as it traverses the right heart. Record the pressures obtained from each location and the systemic arterial blood pressure.

A: Right atrial pressure trace in sinus rhythm. Atrial pressure is clearly lower than that of RV or PA. The 'a' wave coincides with atrial contraction while the 'v' wave reflects atrial filling against the tricuspid valve (closed during RV systole). The 'a' wave will be absent in atrial fibrillation. Large 'v' waves are indicative of tricuspid incompetence.

B: The right ventricular pressure trace is characterized by large swings in pressure that correspond to RV contraction and relaxation.

C: In the PA, the systolic should be equal to RV systolic (in the absence of right ventricular outflow tract obstruction or pulmonary stenosis). Note the dicrotic notch corresponding to closure of the pulmonary valve.

D: Pulmonary capillary wedge pressure. With the PA catheter balloon inflated, the distal port is insulated from the right heart and it is effectively exposed to left atrial pressure. In the absence of pulmonary embolism or pre-capillary pulmonary hypertension then PA diastolic pressure should approximate closely to PCWP.

Fig. 2.7 PA catheter tracing. Reproduced with permission from Myerson SG, Choudhury RP, and Mitchell ARJ (eds) (2010). *Emergencies in Cardiology* (2nd edn). Oxford University Press, Oxford.

Respiratory assessment

Respiratory assessment involves inspection, palpation, percussion, and auscultation, including checking the airway for signs of partial or total obstruction, and an assessment of the chest and breathing. Changes in the respiratory rate are particularly important in identifying those patients who are becoming unwell.

Inspection

- Observe the rate, rhythm, and depth of the patient's breathing. The normal respiratory rate is 12–20 breaths/min.
- Observe for chest symmetry.
- Observe the patient for use of accessory muscles.
- Look for tracheal alignment and scars, e.g. from thoracotomy, sternotomy, or chest drains.
- Look for signs of peripheral (nail beds and earlobes) and central (oral mucosa) cyanosis.
- Check the hands for signs of clubbing (loss of nail-bed angle, ↑ curvature of nail and bulbous ends of fingers).
- Look for signs of spinal curvature, e.g. kyphosis (anteroposterial curvature) or scoliosis (lateral curvature).
- Observe the position of the patient.

Palpation

- Feel the base of the lungs for expansion, which is normally bilateral.
- Check for any signs of surgical oedema (crackling of skin when touched).

Percussion

- Use the fingers to percuss the chest. Work from one side to the other, from the apex to the base of the lungs.
- Normal resonance has a moderately low pitch.
- Hyper-resonance is louder and lower pitched. The causes of hyper-resonance include asthma, COPD, pneumothorax, and emphysema.
- Hyporesonance produces a dull or flat sound. The causes of hypo-resonance include tumours, atelectasis, pneumonia, and pleural effusion.

Auscultation

- Listen for unusual noises—gurgling and snoring could indicate partial airway obstruction.
- Listen for stridor, wheeze (inspiratory and expiratory), and noisy breathing.
- Listen to breath sounds (📖 Breath sounds, p.59).

Also record SaO_2 (📖 Pulse oximetry, p.61). In some instances, arterial blood gases (ABG) (📖 Arterial blood gases, p.62) are required.
   Assess the patient for the following:

- Sputum production.
- Colour and consistency of sputum, if present. Yellow or green sputum could indicate an infection, whereas white, frothy sputum is usually indicative of pulmonary oedema. Blood-stained sputum could be indicative of a PE or lung tumour.

- Shortness of breath and exercise tolerance.
- Does the patient have difficulty in breathing at night?
- Number of pillows required for sleep.
- History of cough—if present, assess presentation (e.g. productive or dry cough).
- Smoking history.
- Can the patient talk with ease?
- Factors precipitating shortness of breath (e.g. cold, exercise, and eating).
- Does the patient have a history of respiratory disease (e.g. lung cancer, COPD, asthma)?

Breath sounds

Comprehensively assessing and interpreting breath sounds is an important skill for any nurse who cares for cardiac patients. Compare both sides of the body because abnormal findings are often restricted to one side, e.g. pneumothorax.

Ideally, the patient should take deep breaths in and out through their mouth while the nurse listens systematically across and down the anterior and posterior of the chest with a stethoscope. As a rule, the sound ↑ in level and pitch as the size of the airway ↑. Auscultate the upper lobes in the anterior chest and the top one-quarter of the posterior fields; the lower lobes take up the bottom three-quarters of the posterior fields. The right middle lobe is heard in the right axilla and the lingula is heard in left axilla. Classify breath sounds as vesicular, bronchial, or added sounds.

Vesicular breath sounds

These are heard over the normal peripheral lung fields during inspiration and the first part of expiration. They are described as having a gentle, low-pitched 'rustling' quality. The sound diminishes in conditions that cause airway obstruction, which limits how the quality of the sound is transmitted through the airways, e.g. asthma or emphysema.

Bronchial breath sounds

Bronchial breathing typically occurs on inspiration and expiration, with a gap in between. An abnormality is present if the sound is heard anywhere other than over the manubrium (top of the sternum). The bronchial breath sound is turbulent and hollow and is similar to the tracheal sound, i.e. harsh, loud, and high in pitch. Bronchial breathing in cardiac patients mainly has the following causes:
• Consolidation
• Upper lobe collapse or atelectasis.

Added sounds

Crackles

▶ Note the timing, location, and intensity of the crackle to determine the underlying cause. Note that pulmonary oedema affects both lungs equally.
• Fine crackles usually occur at the end of inspiration—causes include LVF and pneumonia. If required, respiratory intervention could include noninvasive ventilation (NIV), continuous positive airway pressure (CPAP), or bi-level positive airway pressure (BiPAP).
• Medium crackles heard at the end of inspiration and the beginning of expiration mean that fluid or secretions are present in the bronchioles. Physiotherapist-assisted coughing can help patients expectorate secretions following cardiac surgery.
• Coarse crackles heard throughout respiration usually mean that secretions are present in the main bronchi. They can often be cleared with a cough or 'huff', but some patients might need further intervention, e.g. suctioning if the patient has a tracheostomy.
• Can be caused by pulmonary oedema.

Wheeze

A wheeze heard mainly on expiration is a 'tuneful' note, as air is forced through narrowed airways (e.g. in asthma, COPD, and the presence of a foreign body or tumour). If airflow rates are too low, a wheeze might not be audible.

Stridor

This is usually audible without a stethoscope and indicates a serious obstruction of the large airways. For example, patients who have a tracheostomy following cardiac surgery are at risk of airway occlusion from the build-up of secretions. It is a high-pitched noise normally heard on inspiration.

Rub

This sound is caused by the inflamed pleura rubbing together. The sound could be linked to localized pain and is heard on both inspiration and expiration. Conditions such as pneumonia, pleural effusion, and PE can all cause a pleural rub. It is often described as a low-pitched grating noise like two pieces of leather being rubbed together.

Vocal sounds

Bronchophany

A sound clearly transmitted through a consolidated area, such as infection, collapse, or tumour, is a bronchophany. Ask the patients to say the number '99'; the auscultated sound is clear and loud because there is better sound transmission through 'solid' lung.

Egophany ('e to a')

Commonly heard directly over an area of pleural effusion because of an associated atelectasis of the lung. When auscultated, the sound 'e' becomes a nasal 'a'.

Pulse oximetry

Pulse oximetry provides a noninvasive method of monitoring SpO_2 levels, either continuously or intermittently. It is widely used in both pre-hospital and hospital settings. The normal SpO_2 is >95%. Indications for use include the following:

- Critical illness
- Hypoxia
- Baseline observation
- During surgery
- Post surgery
- Sedation
- Trauma.

Place the probe on the patient's finger or earlobe. If SpO_2 is monitored continuously, the nurse must change the position of the probe regularly to prevent the formation of pressure ulcers and finger stiffness. If the fingers are used, remove nail polish or anything else that may cause problems with the analysis such as blood, paint, grime. Set the monitor alarms. Avoid placing the BP cuff on the same arm as the probe as this will interrupt the readings. The following can lead to inaccurate readings:

- Anaemia
- Jaundice
- SpO_2 <85%
- Poor peripheral perfusion
- Hypothermia
- Rhythm problems
- Nail polish and extensions
- Carbon monoxide poisoning
- Excessive movement, e.g. shivering
- Damaged equipment.

Do not consider SpO_2 levels in isolation, but also consider the clinical presentation. In some cases ABG will need to be obtained (📖 Arterial blood gases, p.62).

Arterial blood gases

ABG measures the level of O_2 and CO_2 in the blood and the acid–base balance within the body. It can also be used to measure sodium and potassium levels. ABG can be measured either through an arterial stab or in the presence of an arterial line, by taking an arterial sample. The procedure for taking a sample from an arterial line is as follows:

- Wash and dry hands. Put on clean gloves.
- Close the three-way tap 'to air', until the syringe is connected. Clean the port of the injectable bung. Connect syringe, turn three-way tap 'on' and collect a 5mL sample of blood from the line.
- Discard this sample and collect a further sample in a pre-heparinized syringe. Turn the three-way tap off.
- Using the flush device flush the line and then the bung on the port (attach a syringe).
- Take the sample to the blood gas machine and follow the manufacturer's instructions.

Normal values

The normal values are as follows:
- pH 7.35–7.45
- pO_2 10.1–13.9kPa
- pCO_2 4.0–6kPa
- Bicarbonate (HCO_3) 22–26mmol/L
- Base excess (BE) –2 to +2.

To interpret the ABG, use the following process:
- Look at the pO_2: although this does not affect the acid–base balance as such, it indicates hypoxia. ▶ Take account of any O_2 therapy that the patient is receiving.
- Look at the pH: if pH is <7.35 = acidosis; pH >7.45 = alkalosis.
- Look at the pCO_2: pCO_2 <4.0kPa can indicate respiratory alkalosis; pCO_2 >6.0kPa can indicate respiratory acidosis (see Table 2.5).
- Look at the HCO_3: ↑ HCO_3 can indicate metabolic alkalosis; ↓ HCO_3 can indicate metabolic acidosis.
- Look at the BE: ↑ BE indicates metabolic alkalosis; ↓ BE indicates metabolic acidosis.

The following are some of the causes of respiratory acidosis (high CO_2):
- Type 2 respiratory failure
- Effects of sedatives
- Head injury
- Inadequate ventilation
- Pulmonary oedema.

The following are some of the causes of respiratory alkalosis:
- Hyperventilation
- Wrong ventilator settings.

The following are some of the causes of metabolic acidosis:
- Renal failure
- Diabetic ketoacidosis (DKA)
- Shock
- Cardiac arrest.

The following are some of the causes of metabolic alkalosis:
- Overdose of antacids
- Severe vomiting.

Compensation

In the case of metabolic acidosis or alkalosis, compensation takes place by a change in respiratory rate. If the patient is metabolically acidotic, the respiratory rate ↑; ∴, blowing off CO_2 and H_2O causing the pH to become less acid. Alternatively, if the cause of the problem is respiratory, the kidneys either retain or secrete more hydrogen ions to compensate. However, this mechanism takes some time.

Table 2.5 Effects of acidosis and alkalosis on pH, $PaCO_2$, and HCO_3

	pH	$PaCO_2$	HCO_3
Respiratory acidosis	↓	↑	N
Respiratory alkalosis	↑	↓	N
Respiratory acidosis with compensation	↓N	↑	↑
Respiratory alkalosis with compensation	↑N	↓	↓
Metabolic acidosis	↓	N	↓
Metabolic alkalosis	↑	N	↑
Metabolic acidosis with compensation	↓N	↓	↓
Metabolic alkalosis with compensation	↑N	↑	↑
Mixed acidosis	↓	↑	↓

↓, decreased; ↑, increased; N, normal.

Chest X-ray (CXR)

Use the CXR in conjunction with the findings of inspection, percussion, palpation, and auscultation. CXR are taken from anterior–posterior ('mobile'), posterior–anterior ('standard'), or lateral perspectives. This section does not include interpretation of lateral CXR. The majority of nurses recognize standard and mobile CXR, the latter is common in critical care areas, where patients are often too sick to have a standard CXR. ▶ Nurses should be familiar with what is 'normal' on the CXR so they can quickly refer any suspected 'abnormal' presentation for appropriate medical or physiotherapist interpretation and intervention.

Basic interpretation

- Check the patient's name and the date are correct on the viewing screen and step back.
- Note the patient's age and gender, because this could help exclude or support a diagnosis (e.g. are there breast shadows?). Notice mastectomy.
- Examine the presentation of the film: decide if it is anterior–posterior (marked) or posterior–anterior (unmarked). ▶ The heart appears larger on an anterior–posterior film.
- Orientation: check the radiographer's 'left' and 'right' markings; the heart is not always on the left, it can be repositioned (e.g. by tension pneumothorax or dextrocardia).
- If the film is anterior–posterior, is the film marked 'erect' or 'supine'? (Fluid levels might not be apparent on a supine film.)
- Is there rotation? If the patient's position is rotated, one lung might appear to be whiter.
- Penetration: the vertebrae should only just be visible through the lower part of the cardiac shadow.
- Check the degree of inspiration: poor inspiratory effort makes the heart appear larger and gives an appearance of basal shadowing and right-tracheal deviation.
- Systematically examine the film in its entirety, noting any abnormalities. In a posterior–anterior film the normal cardiothoracic ratio should be <0.5.
- Identify the location of the abnormality, e.g. heart, lungs, or pleura, and describe its appearance, e.g. too white, too dark, an abnormal size, or in the wrong place.
- Always link your findings to your assessment of the patient: do they confirm what you heard on percussion or auscultation (▢ Respiratory assessment, p.57)?

Abnormalities on CXR

There are a number of cardiac-related abnormalities that can be identified on CXR.

Left ventricular failure

- Upper lobe blood diversion (early sign). ▶ Only significant on an 'erect' film.
- Kerley B lines—indicate pulmonary oedema. They are small horizontal lines that are best seen at the lung peripheries, above the costophrenic angle.
- A 'Bat's wing' appearance as alveolar shadows radiate from the hila with severe pulmonary oedema. There may be hazier shadowing throughout the lungs and noticeable air bronchograms.
- ↑ cardiothoracic ratio—left ventricular dilatation is highly likely to be caused by heart failure. ❶ With acute onset of LVF, there might be no cardiac enlargement.

Mitral stenosis

- LA enlargement causes the appearance of the left heart border to change from concave to straight, or even bulge outwards.
- The left main bronchus is elevated because of LA enlargement (i.e. the angle between the carina and bronchi is >90°).
- There might be a 'double' shadow at the right heart border caused by LA dilation. The right heart border can also appear more towards the right than normal.
- There is upper lobe blood diversion because of ↑ LA pressure and Kerley B lines might result from interstitial oedema.
- Rarely, there is visible calcification (dense whiteness) in the area of the MV.

Pericardial effusion

- A sudden, ↑ size/cardiothoracic ratio on the posterior–anterior film.
- Generalized enlargement of the heart shadow, which is bulbous in shape and can cover both hila.
- The vascular markings across the lung fields are usually normal.
- The superior vena cava might be engorged (↑ tracheal density to the right edge >3mm) on an 'erect' CXR.

Left ventricular aneurysm

- ↑ cardiothoracic ratio on posterior–anterior CXR.
- A prominent, outwards left ventricular 'bulge' is visible along the left heart border.
- In severe cases, there might be associated signs of pulmonary oedema/ LVF.
- Calcification can occur along the edge of the left heart border if the aneurysm has existed for a long time—this aspect can also occur in other disease processes, e.g. tuberculosis.

Consolidation

- Can be difficult to diagnose—check whether the patient has signs of infection, e.g. pyrexia, sputum, and cough.
- The alveolar spaces are filled with fluid that appears 'white' on the CXR—note whether the small airways are visible (black) as air bronchograms within the white areas.
- Fluid sinks, so the 'whiteness' of consolidation becomes denser as it moves lower down the lung.
- Consolidation is usually a temporary occurrence so comparison of the patient's CXRs can exclude any chronic alternative, such as fibrosis.
- If the whiteness has clearly marked borders and is uniformly dense in appearance, it is more likely to be an area of lung collapse or a pleural effusion.

Pneumothorax

- Absence of normal vascular lung markings, making the lung field appear 'black'. Note: bullous disease is unlikely if the rest of the lung fields appear normal. Lung markings crossing or peripheral to an area of blackness are more likely to indicate a bulla.
- Check if there is a visible 'lung edge'—this is not normally seen. Look at the upper zones as air is more likely to accumulate here. It may be useful to turn the CXR on its side as this can help identify the lung edge more clearly.
- Identify any mediastinal shift—movement away from the black area can indicate a tension pneumothorax (medical emergency).

Visible cardiac devices on CXR

The following devices and prostheses can be highly visible on the CXR and used to confirm a history if the patient is unable to do so or support a diagnosis, e.g. incorrect positioning of a pacing wire (e.g. tamponade or failure to capture) or a poorly positioned chest drain (e.g. surgical emphysema or kinking):

- Permanent pacemaker box—usually underneath left clavicle, with visible pacing wires. Clearly identify whether the wires are atrial or ventricular, or both.
- Temporary pacing wire—coiled externally, often sited in a subclavian vein, and positioned distally towards the apex of the right ventricle.
- Mechanical prosthetic valves—depending on the positioning, the ball-and-cage or tilting-disc mechanism might be clearly identifiable.
- Valvular annuloplasty ring.
- A central line or PA catheter—commonly through the subclavian or internal jugular vein.
- Sternal wires—after cardiac surgery, e.g. CABG or valve replacement.
- External ECG wires, clips, and electrodes.
- Epicardial pacing wires.
- Chest drains—either pleural or mediastinal. Identify apical and basal placement of pleural drains.
- Pigtail catheter—from pericardiocentesis after pericardial effusion.
- Implantable cardioverter defibrillator (ICD).

Related guidance

Moya A, Sutton R, Ammirati F, Blanc J, et al. (2009) Guidelines for the diagnosis and management of syncope (vers09) Task Force for the diagnosis and management of syncope of the European Society of Cardiology. *European Heart Journal* **30**, 2631–71.

Westby M, Davis S, Bullock I, et al. (2010) *Transient Loss of Consciousness ("Blackouts") Management in Adults and Young People*. National Clinical Guideline Centre for Acute and Chronic Conditions, Royal College of Physicians, London.

Cardiac investigations

Introduction

There are numerous invasive and noninvasive tests used in the diagnosis of cardiac disease. Most of the tests are performed by specialist operators in suitably equipped laboratories. However, it is useful for nurses working with patients with suspected or diagnosed cardiac disease to have a broad understanding of the main diagnostic tests available. See also Chapter 2 (📖 Cardiac monitoring, p.41; 12-Lead electrocardiogram (ECG), p.43) for discussion of ECG, Chapter 8 (📖 Coronary angiography: preprocedure care, p.139) for discussion of coronary angiography, and Chapter 13 for a discussion of electrophysiology studies.

Exercise tolerance testing

The exercise tolerance test (ETT) is based on the premise that the ECG shows ischaemic changes (ST-segment depression) when patients with CHD exercise. ETTs are noninvasive, relatively cheap, and reasonably easy to perform. It should be noted that false-negative and false-positive tests are obtained in some cases and, as with other cardiac investigations, the results should be interpreted in the light of other available data.

Exercise testing has the following indications:
- Evaluation of chest pain and diagnosis of CHD
- Evaluation of arrhythmias
- Stratification of high-risk patients—to determine the course of treatment
- Evaluation of prognosis and treatment post-MI
- Evaluation of treatment and cardiac function pre and post revascularization
- Assessment of cardiopulmonary function in patients with dilated cardiomyopathy or heart failure.

Exercise testing is contraindicated in patients with the following conditions:
- Obvious heart failure
- Unstable angina, acute MI, or known severe LMS stenosis
- Severe AS
- Uncontrolled hypertension
- Significant arrhythmia at rest
- Acute myocarditis or pericarditis
- Recent aortic surgery or dissecting aortic aneurysm
- Fever.

The test involves exercising the patient on a treadmill or stationary bicycle, while simultaneously monitoring ECG, HR, and BP. Patients should be advised not to eat ≤1h before the test, because this could affect their performance. β-blockers are usually discontinued the day before the test and digoxin is discontinued a week before the test. The exercise protocol varies, but the Bruce protocol is the most widely used as it has been extensively validated. Normally, 3–4 stages, each lasting 3min, are used. A modified Bruce protocol is used for testing patients within 1wk of an acute MI. The patient always starts on a low level of exercise, which then gradually ↑. As the test progresses, any ECG or BP changes that accompany the expected ↑ in HR are noted. The test ends when the patient completes the set exercise protocol, although monitoring continues in the recovery period after the exercise. The test is terminated if the patient experiences progressively worsening symptoms of ischaemia (e.g. angina, faintness, dyspnoea, or haemodynamic instability) during the exercise test. Full resuscitation facilities must be in the vicinity. The test usually takes ~20min in total.

The ETT has been associated with diagnostic and prognostic limitations, particularly in relation to sensitivity (the ability to detect coronary artery disease [CAD]) and specificity (the ability to exclude those without CAD). Its use has been questioned in certain patient groups including women, the elderly, and specific ethnic groups. The ETT is currently being phased out in favour of CT calcium scoring; the aforementioned limitations being major contributing factors.

Ambulatory monitoring

Ambulatory electrocardiography (AECG) allows monitoring of patients while they carry out their normal activities. It is often used to determine the cause of intermittent symptoms thought to be due to a cardiac arrhythmia and is indicated for patients with the following conditions:

- Suspected bradyarrhythmias
- Suspected tachyarrhythmias
- Evaluation of pharmacological treatment in patients with established arrhythmias.

AECG may be achieved by a Holter monitor or a patient-activated device (event recorder). A Holter monitor is a small lightweight device which requires the attachment of electrodes to the patient's chest; these devices enable continuous recording of the ECG for up to a week, possibly longer, ↑ the likelihood of capturing a symptomatic arrhythmia. The data retrieved is interpreted retrospectively and cannot be viewed in real time.

If the patient's symptoms are infrequent, Holter monitoring may not capture abnormal episodes. In this instance, a patient-activated recorder may be used, whereby the patient can activate a recording at the onset of symptoms, such as palpitations or dizziness.

Patients are asked to keep a note of both activities and symptoms when undergoing AECG monitoring, so that any abnormal readings can be linked to the patient's activity and the presence (or absence) of symptoms. Patients are asked not to touch the electrodes during the monitoring period and to avoid activities such as swimming and showering.

Tilt testing

The tilt test is commonly performed on patients who present with syncope of unknown origin. Syncope is a sudden, transient loss of consciousness, with an accompanying loss of postural tone.

The tilt test is noninvasive and aims to provoke neurally mediated syncope (NMS) (vasovagal syncope) as an aid to diagnosis. It is especially useful before more invasive electrophysiological studies in patients in whom other noninvasive tests are inconclusive. NMS results from a breakdown of the feedback mechanisms between the parasympathetic and sympathetic nervous systems. Under normal circumstances, when an individual assumes an upright position, blood pools in the lower extremities and ↓ arterial pressure. This initiates sympathetic activity, resulting in ↑ HR and BP. In some people, this reflex is overridden by ↑ vagal tone, resulting in vasodilation and ↓ CO, bradycardia, and syncope.

The tilt test is usually performed in an electrophysiology laboratory, with full resuscitation equipment available. The patient also requires IV access for the infusion of fluids and drugs. The test involves strapping the patient to a special tilt table with a footboard. The patient is monitored: first, lying in a supine position; and then, with the table moved to an upright tilt (head up) of 60–80° for 10–60min. The patient's HR, BP, and symptoms (if present) are recorded every 3–5min and the ECG is continuously recorded. The test is positive if any one or more of the following events occur:
• If the patient becomes symptomatic
• ↑ signs of bradycardia
• ↓ BP

Moving the table back to the horizontal position usually reverses the symptoms.

 If the test result is negative, some units perform a second tilt test that includes IV isoprenaline to ↑ the patient's HR when they are supine. However, this drug is contraindicated in those with CHD.

Treatment for NMS varies depending on exact symptoms, but includes education on recognition of prodromal symptoms, pharmacological therapy, and pacing. These mostly reduce symptoms rather than prevent attacks.

Imaging studies: echocardiography

Rapid advances in technology have expanded the portfolio of imaging techniques used to diagnose cardiac patients and evaluate treatment. A variety of methods aid visualization of the heart and its abnormalities (if any). All of these imaging studies can be carried out on an out-patient basis, although they are also used on in-patients. It is important to explain the procedure to the patient so that they know what to expect, and it is also important to schedule follow-up appointments so that the results, and any subsequent changes with treatment, can be discussed. The choice of imaging study depends on the severity and presentation of the patient's symptoms and on its availability.

Echocardiography

Echocardiography (commonly abbreviated to 'Echo' in clinical practice) is an important diagnostic imaging tool in cardiology, which uses ultrasound technology. It is the most commonly used investigative test after ECG recording. The imaging process involves directing ultrasound waves at the chest using a transducer and analysing the rebounding waves from the heart's walls and valves using a computer to calculate the size, shape, and movement of structures in the heart. This information is mapped to pixels and displayed on-screen as a visual image, which can be stored digitally. Echo does not produce pictures with a resolution that is high enough to see arteries, but it does identify abnormalities in heart structure and function (e.g. incompetent valves, akinetic walls, and thrombi in the heart chambers). Echo is especially useful in determining left ventricular function.

Technological advances mean that two-dimensional (2D), three-dimensional (3D), and Doppler Echo are available. 3D Echo provides additional information to the standard Echo and allows improved assessment of ventricular volumes and improved detection of a thrombus within the left atrial appendage. Doppler Echo provides information about blood flow and is particularly useful in quantifying valve anomalies and turbulent blood flow. ↑ use of stress Echo has enhanced the accuracy of standard exercise testing. Stress Echo involves comparing baseline images with those taken at peak exercise and can identify abnormal stress response such as ↓ in ventricular wall thickening or ↓ wall motion. A contrast Echo refers to the administration of an IV injection of an ultrasound contrast agent containing albumin microbubbles. It is often referred to as a 'bubble study'. Contrast Echo has a role in the diagnosis of shunts including atrial septal defect (ASD) and patent foramen ovale (PFO).

The advantages of Echo are as follows:
• Noninvasive
• Relatively quick
• Requires minimal patient preparation
• Portable—for use in a variety of settings.

Transthoracic echocardiography (TTE)

TTE is the most common form of Echo. The patient needs to remove clothing from the upper half of their body; advise the patient that a gel is applied to the transducer/probe, which is then moved across their chest. The test also requires patient cooperation with breathing and positioning. There is no specific postinvestigation care.

Transoesophageal echocardiography (TOE)

TOE is semi-invasive, because the transducer is mounted on an endoscope and passed orally into the oesophagus. The transducer sits adjacent to the posterior aspect of the heart, which gives a better image resolution than TTE.

TOE is indicated as follows:
• When TTE has not provided diagnostic information.
• To aid in the diagnosis of IE.
• To rule out atrial thrombus before cardioversion.
• To identify abnormalities after unexplained stroke or systemic emboli.
• To confirm suspected aortic dissection or atrial mass.
• To assess mitral valve function.
• To monitor myocardial function during some types of surgery (e.g. cardiac surgery or surgery on patients with cardiac problems).

Although unit protocols vary, ensure the patient fasts for 4h before the investigation because of the risk of aspiration. Dentures should be removed. The patient's throat is anaesthetized and conscious sedation is required because the patient needs to cooperate to swallow the endoscope. During the procedure, record ECG continuously and monitor arterial oxygen saturation (SaO_2); record HR and BP frequently. Airway management is vital and frequent oral suction is required throughout the procedure.

Advise the patient to wait for 1h after TOE before eating and drinking, to allow the local anaesthetic to wear off.

Imaging studies: nuclear and cardiac magnetic resonance

Nuclear cardiology

Use of radioisotope tracers is common; however, these studies have a moderate radiation risk, which should be explained to the patient.

Positron emission tomography (PET)

PET uses nuclear imaging to determine myocardial viability in patients with impaired left ventricular function resulting from CAD. A short-lived tracer of blood flow is used in combination with a metabolic imager, which differentiates between normal, infarcted, and hibernating myocardium. It is especially useful for determining which patients could benefit from revascularization.

PET is relatively expensive and, ∴, is mainly used as a research application.

Myocardial perfusion scintigraphy (MPS)

MPS (also known as single-photon emission computerized tomography [SPECT]) involves intravenously injecting the patient with a radioisotope that is taken up by the myocardium. The isotope gives off γ-rays that are detected by a computerized scintillation camera, which then produces an image showing the concentration of the isotope in a particular area of the heart (scintigraphy). SPECT images are displayed as a series of consecutive slices through the heart. The isotopes are usually injected while the patient exercises on a treadmill; however, patients who cannot exercise adequately are given pharmacological agents (e.g. adenosine or dipyridamole) by IV infusion to stress the heart. Images of the stressed heart are compared with those taken after the heart has rested for 2–4h. Thallium-201 (hence the name 'thallium scan') and technetium (TC-sestamibi) are the most commonly used isotopes.

The isotope is taken up by viable myocardium and thus hypoperfused areas show up as 'cold spots' on the scan. Cold spots that appear on exercise imaging but not on imaging at rest indicate reversible or exercise-induced ischaemia, and cold spots that appear on both sets of images suggest infarction. However, thallium scans cannot distinguish between old and new infarcts.

MPS is indicated as follows:

- To assess whether coronary obstruction is present in patients with suspected coronary disease.
- To guide revascularization in those with known coronary disease.
- To assess adequacy of revascularization.
- To determine the probability of further events.
- SPECT is recommended as the initial diagnostic tool for people with suspected coronary disease in whom ETT poses problems of poor sensitivity or difficulties of interpretation.

Radionuclide ventriculography

Also known as a multiple-gated acquisition (MUGA) scan. This scan studies the working action of the heart and is most often used post MI.

An IV injection of technetium-99 is given. Radioactivity is measured in the heart during the cardiac cycle. Using these measurements a computer calculates the ejection fraction. Arrhythmias (e.g. AF), which have beat-to-beat filling and cycle-length differentials, ↓ the accuracy of the calculation. There is no special preparation or aftercare with this type of scan.

Cardiac magnetic resonance (CMR) imaging

CMR uses a strong magnetic field to produce a 3D image of the body and is useful in any condition affecting the heart. Magnetic resonance imaging (MRI) is particularly useful in monitoring patients with aortic dissections and cardiac masses, but it can be contraindicated in those who have an implanted cardiac pacemaker or defibrillator because its magnetic field can interfere with their operation (unless they have a model that is MRI safe). Use MRI with caution in patients who have metal prosthetic valves or stents, or those who require intensive haemodynamic monitoring, because there is a minor risk of internal movement and projectile or thermal injury from metallic prostheses or equipment. The use of contrast agents differentiates between ischaemic and infarcted myocardium and so it is useful for those with equivocal ETT results. However, CMR is expensive and not widely available so its use is currently limited. There is no particular preparation for CMR, although warn patients that it involves lying still in a tight 'tube', which may produce feelings of claustrophobia.

Imaging studies: computed tomography calcium scoring

Over time atherosclerotic plaques become calcified. Computed tomography (CT) calcium scoring is a noninvasive test using CT scanning to detect and measure calcium within the coronary arteries. CT uses X-ray absorption data from multiple directions to produce cross-sectional images of the body. The amount of calcium within the coronary arteries is converted to a calcium score which correlates with the severity of the blockage. Interpretation of the scores and recommendations are as follows:[1]

- A score of 0 indicates a negative test; alternative causes of chest pain should be considered.
- A score of <400 indicates that the likelihood of a future coronary event is above average. Further investigation is recommended, e.g. CT coronary angiography.
- A score of >400 indicates that the likelihood of a future coronary event is high. Invasive coronary angiography is recommended.

Following the publication of the NICE guidelines on the assessment and diagnosis of recent onset chest pain,[1] calcium scoring is playing an increasingly important role in the diagnosis, management, and risk stratification of patients with CAD. Patients presenting with chest pain who are thought to be at a low risk of CAD were traditionally offered an ETT. NICE recommend that such patients should be offered CT calcium scoring. In practice this means that hospitals may have to purchase appropriate CT scanners; this could have huge economic implications for the NHS budget. It does, however, offer advantages over ETT to the patient. The procedure is quicker and it has much higher sensitivity for detecting CAD, meaning that fewer patients will be referred for further unnecessary testing.[2]

Related guidance

Department of Health (2011) *A Review of Emerging Cardiac Technologies*. Department of Health, London.

National Institute for Health and Clinical Excellence (2012) *New generation cardiac CT scanners (Aquilion ONE, Brilliance iCT, Discovery CT750 HD and Somatom Definition Flash) for cardiac imaging in people with suspected or known coronary artery disease in whom imaging is difficult with earlier generation CT scanners*. NICE diagnostics guidance 3. NICE, London.

[1] National Institute for Health and Clinical Excellence (2010) *Chest pain of recent onset: assessment and diagnosis of recent onset chest pain or discomfort of suspected cardiac origin*. (NICE Clinical Guideline 95). NICE, London. ℳ http://www.nice.org.uk

[2] National Institute for Health and Clinical Excellence (2010) *Chest pain of recent onset. CT calcium scoring factsheet. Implementing NICE guidance*. (NICE Clinical Guideline 95). NICE, London. ℳ http://www.nice.org.uk

Valvular disease

Introduction

Valvular disorders such as regurgitation or stenosis can affect any of the four heart valves, although they are more likely to cause problems to the valves on the left side of the heart than the right, due to higher pressures on the left side. In many cases the symptoms of valvular disease take many years to develop and may be gradual in onset and severity. Some of the signs and symptoms experienced are related to heart failure and are discussed in Chapter 10. The patient can be managed medically but may eventually require valve replacement or repair. Over the last few years newer techniques have been developed for replacing or repairing valves. This chapter covers the causes, signs and symptoms, and management of valvular disorders. Table 4.1 provides a comparison of the signs and symptoms of the different types of valvular problems on the left side of the heart.

Table 4.1 Signs and symptoms of valve disease

Mitral stenosis	Mitral regurgitation	Aortic stenosis	Aortic regurgitation
AF	AF	Dyspnoea	Fatigue
Cough at night	Cough at night	Fatigue	Diastolic murmur
Haemoptysis	Shortness of breath on exertion (SOBOE)	Palpitations	Widened arterial pulse pressure
Fatigue	↑ HR	Syncope	
Symptoms of RHF—peripheral oedema, abdominal ascites	↓ BP	Angina	Palpitations
	Symptoms of RHF	Ejection systolic murmur	
Paroxysmal nocturnal dyspnoea (PND)	Fatigue	Conduction problems	
Malar flush		Late AF	
Mid diastolic murmur		SOBOE	
P mitrale on ECG			

Aortic stenosis

The aortic valve lies between the aorta and left ventricle. It has three leaflets or cusps, which are closed in diastole and open in systole. The normal size of the valve orifice is 3–4cm^2.

Aetiology

Aortic stenosis (AS) is one of the commonest acquired valvular lesions, occurring in 2–7% of those aged >65yrs. The normal aortic valve has three leaflets (cusps); however, some people are born with bicuspid aortic valves.

Causes

- Calcification (♂ sex, age, and hypercholesterolaemia are all predisposing factors).
- Degeneration of the valve.
- Congenital bicuspid valve.
- Stenosis occurring above or below the aortic ring (supravalvular and subvalvular, respectively).
- Rheumatic fever (rare).

The narrowed aortic valve leads to left ventricular hypertrophy (LVH) and LV dilatation. This will eventually lead to LV failure with a ↓ in CO and ejection fraction (EF). Eventually, the patient may develop pulmonary hypertension and right-sided heart failure.

Signs and symptoms

Symptoms do not usually appear for many years. The symptoms experienced depend on the degree of stenosis and LV dysfunction. Patients who have a previous history of rheumatic fever may also have mitral stenosis (MS), and this will usually present first. Common signs and symptoms of AS include the following:

- Tiredness.
- Palpitations.
- Syncope occurs in ~25% of patients, particularly during exercise.
- Angina (due to ↑ O$_2$ demand from LVH and possible ↓ supply). Angina is more common in AS than in any other valve disorder.
- Dyspnoea (most common symptom).
- Murmur—ejection systolic murmur.
- Conduction problems—the calcification process may affect the bundle of His.
- May have ↓ BP
- Atrial fibrillation (AF) is a late sign, which indicates a poor prognosis.

Diagnosis

- ECG—LVH pattern. Left-axis deviation and left bundle branch block (LBBB) may also be present.
- Echocardiogram—appearance of valve cusps (i.e. thickening or calcification), presence of LVH and left ventricular outflow tract obstruction (LVOTO) can be assessed. The gradient across the valve can be measured: normal gradient is <20mmHg and severe gradient is >60mmHg.

- CXR—LVH, dilated aorta, and pulmonary congestion.
- Cardiac catheter—presence of CAD can be established. The gradient can be measured if the stenosis is not too severe.
- Exercise tolerance test—only in asymptomatic patients to identify exercise-induced haemodynamic compromise.

Management

Management will depend on symptoms. This may include β-blockers to ↓ myocardial O_2 demand. Statins and ACE inhibitors may be used to slow the progression of the disease and improve death rates from cardiovascular events. Patients with AS need a high preload to maintain a satisfactory CO. Medication that can ↓ preload, such as nitrates and diuretics, must, ∴, be used with caution. Patients who have a critical stenosis should avoid vigorous exercise (a severe stenosis is defined as aortic valve orifice of <0.7cm²). Aortic valve replacement surgery is usually the first line of treatment once symptoms have developed because of poor prognosis. However transcatheter aortic valve implantation (TAVI) (📖 Transcatheter aortic valve implantation (TAVI or TAVR), p.91) can now be used particularly for those patients not suitable for open heart surgery.

Aortic regurgitation

Aetiology

Aortic regurgitation (AR) leads to a leakage of blood from the aorta into the LV during diastole. Diseases that affect the aortic root or valve leaflets cause AR. If AR has been caused by rheumatic fever, it can also be associated with MS and AS. AR can be acute or chronic depending on the cause.

Causes

- Rheumatic fever (rare)—leaflets become thickened and fused
- IE
- Dilatation of the aortic root (e.g. syphilis, Marfan's syndrome, or dissecting aortic aneurysm)
- Trauma
- Degenerative changes
- Congenital bicuspid valve.

Regurgitation through the aortic valve leads to LV dilatation and, eventually, LVH and failure. This may result in chest pain. In time, the lungs may be affected, with pulmonary congestion developing.

Signs and symptoms

As with AS, in chronic AR symptoms may not appear for many years. Once LV function starts to deteriorate the patient will develop shortness of breath (which is the main presenting feature in both acute and chronic cases). Other signs and symptoms include the following:

- Tiredness
- Chest pain—less common in AR than AS
- Palpitations
- Widened arterial pulse pressure
- High-pitched (diastolic) murmur.

If AR is acute compensatory mechanisms will not have had time to develop and the patient may present with ↑ P, ↓ BP, and cardiogenic shock.

Diagnosis

- ECG—LVH and left atrial hypertrophy (LAH) may be present.
- Echo—LV function assessed. Doppler Echo is better as it shows the size of the aortic orifice.
- TOE—aortic dissection may be viewed.
- CXR—cardiac enlargement.
- Cardiac catheter—LV dysfunction, coronary artery anatomy and degree of regurgitation.

Management

Patients with mild or moderate AR are commonly asymptomatic and will not usually require surgery. Assessment of symptoms, ECG, and imaging (echocardiogram and CXR) will be performed every 6–12 months. Diuretics may be used to improve shortness of breath. ACE inhibitors can be used for LV dilatation. High diastolic BP needs to be controlled. β-blockers and other drugs that ↓ LV function and prolong diastole are usually contraindicated because this will ↑ regurgitation. Inotropes may be required for acute AR. Aortic valve replacement surgery is usually considered once patients develop symptoms, particularly if they are consistent with New York Heart Association (NYHA) class III or IV (￼ Classification of heart failure, p.197), or in asymptomatic patients with EF <50%.

Mitral valve prolapse

The mitral valve (MV) lies between the LA and LV. It has two leaflets that are supported by chordae tendineae and papillary muscles. The normal size of the mitral valve orifice is 4–5cm². The mitral valve must remain closed during systole; ∴, this valve is under significantly more pressure than the aortic valve.

Aetiology

Mitral valve prolapse (MVP) is the most common valve disorder; 25–50% of cases are hereditary, and it primarily affects young ♀. It can progress to mitral valve regurgitation (MR).

Causes

- Hereditary
- Marfan's syndrome.

Signs and symptoms

Often symptomless, but then similar symptoms to MR develop. Symptoms may appear transiently.

Common signs and symptoms of MVP include the following:

- Tiredness
- Anxiety—due to knowledge of condition
- Palpitations—from ↑ sinus rate
- Dizziness and syncope
- Shortness of breath
- Heart murmur—late systolic murmur
- Nonspecific chest pain.

Diagnosis

- ECG—usually normal, unless MR present
- Echocardiogram
- TOE—indicates whether chordal rupture has occurred
- CXR—often normal.

Management

Reassurance and follow-up, but otherwise no treatment, unless MR develops.

Mitral valve regurgitation

Aetiology
Mitral valve regurgitation (MR) leads to a leakage of blood between the LV and LA during systole.

Causes
- Degenerative changes.
- Ischaemic heart disease—the papillary muscle may be damaged as a result of acute MI.
- Chordal rupture—more common in ♂ than ♀. Can be caused by fibrosis of the papillary muscle or MI.
- Trauma to leaflets.
- LA myxoma.
- IE—may damage the leaflets or the chordae tendineae.
- Calcification—occurs more commonly in ♀. AS may also be present.
- Hypertrophic obstructive cardiomyopathy.
- MVP.

Signs and symptoms
Regurgitation through the mitral valve leads to ↑ LV volume at the end of diastole (preload) and ↓ afterload because of regurgitation back to the LA. ↑ preload and ↓ afterload means that a larger volume of blood should be ejected from the LV; however, because some blood goes back into the LA, CO ↓. Initially, the heart will compensate for this by LV dilatation and LVH but, eventually, the LV will fail.

LA dilatation can lead to ↑ pulmonary venous pressure. In time, the pressure in the pulmonary artery will ↑, leading to right-sided heart failure. In chronic MR, symptoms may not develop for many years. However, in acute MR, the patient will experience acute shortness of breath as a result of a sudden ↑ in pulmonary venous pressure.

Common signs and symptoms of MR include the following:
- AF—due to enlargement of the LA; ~1/3 of patients with MR will develop AF
- Cough at night
- Shortness of breath—at night and on exertion
- ↑ HR and ↓ BP
- Fatigue
- Symptoms of right-sided heart failure (e.g. peripheral oedema and abdominal distension).

Diagnosis
- ECG—LVH, LAH, and AF
- Echocardiogram—assess LV function, valve size, and shape and degree of regurgitation
- CXR—LAH and LVH.

Management

The patient will be treated according to their symptoms (i.e. diuretics and vasodilators for biventricular failure). A grading system may be used to assess the severity of symptoms and help determine treatment options. Hypertension needs to be controlled because this can lead to ↑ regurgitation. The mitral valve may be repaired or replaced surgically. AF or LV problems (e.g. EF <0.60, NYHA class II) are a good indicator that surgery is required. Percutaneous techniques such as MitraClip® (📖 Percutaneous mitral valve repair, p.91) can be used for patients who are not suitable for surgery.

Mitral valve stenosis

Aetiology

Mitral stenosis (MS) ↓ the amount of blood flowing into the LV during diastole. Narrowing of the mitral valve orifice to <2.5cm² leads to ↑ pressure gradient across the valve. MS affects more ♀ than ♂ and is more common in the older adult. MS is less common in Western countries.

Causes

Rheumatic fever—this is the most common cause of MS. The valve leaflets become thickened.

Signs and symptoms

It is normally ~20–40yrs between occurrence of rheumatic fever and the onset of MS symptoms. As the stenosis ↑, the pressure in the LA elevates, which leads to LA dilatation. This will eventually cause pulmonary pressures to ↑, leading to right-sided heart failure.

Common signs and symptoms of MS include the following:
- Shortness of breath—the most common symptom in MS. It is often related to exertion/exercise.
- AF—due to LA enlargement.
- Cough—caused by pulmonary congestion or pressure on the bronchial tree from the enlarged LA.
- Haemoptysis—due to the ↑ pressure in the pulmonary capillaries.
- Fatigue.
- Symptoms of right-sided heart failure (e.g. peripheral oedema and abdominal distension).
- Paroxysmal nocturnal dyspnoea—usually a later symptom.
- Butterfly-wing pattern on cheeks (Malar flush)—due to local cyanosis.
- Murmur—mid-diastolic murmur.
- Infective endocarditis (Chapter 5).

Diagnosis

- ECG—P mitrale (LAH), right-axis deviation, right ventricular hypertrophy (RVH), and AF
- Echo—assess valve movement and leaflets
- CXR—LAH and RVH
- Cardiac catheter—assess CO and diastolic pressure gradient.

Management

Diuretics may be used to ↓ preload and venous congestion. Anticoagulants and antiarrhythmics will be required if AF is present. As with other valve problems, prophylactic antibiotics will be required before any invasive procedure.

A percutaneous valvuloplasty or valve replacement surgery may be performed. Surgery is usually considered when the valve area is <1.5cm² or NYHA class III–IV is present (📖 Classification of heart failure, p.197).

Pulmonary valve disorders

The valves on the right side of the heart are under significantly less pressure than those on the left side. The pulmonary valve sits between the RV and pulmonary artery. It has three leaflets.

Aetiology

Pulmonary valve disorders are usually related to a congenital problem, such as tetralogy of Fallot, and will usually be discovered in infants more commonly than in adults because of the resulting signs and symptoms of the congenital problem.

Causes

- Congenital
- Carcinoma
- IE.

Signs and symptoms

Pulmonary valve disease will lead to right-sided heart failure. The signs and symptoms exhibited will depend on other congenital abnormalities (e.g. LVOTO and ventricular septal defect [VSD]).

Common signs and symptoms of pulmonary valve disorders include the following:

- Peripheral oedema
- Abdominal distension
- Shortness of breath.

Diagnosis

- ECG—RVH
- Echo—the cause of right ventricular outflow tract obstruction (RVOTO; e.g. vegetation) will be seen.

Management

Repair or replacement either percutaneously or open heart surgery.

Tricuspid valve disorders

The tricuspid valve sits between the RA and RV. It has three leaflets or cusps.

Aetiology

Tricuspid valve disease is rare. Tricuspid valve disease may exist in the presence of disease of the mitral valve or aortic valve.

Causes

• Rheumatic fever—rare in developing countries
• Congenital disorders
• Trauma, e.g. pacing wire insertion.

Signs and symptoms

TS causes ↑ pressure in the RA, which leads to RA dilatation, jugular vein distension, heptomegaly, abdominal distension, and oedema.

Tricuspid regurgitation leads to raised venous pressure.

Common signs and symptoms of tricuspid valve disorders include the following:

• Peripheral oedema
• Abdominal distension.

Diagnosis

• ECG—RAH
• Echo—Doppler Echo is better as it shows the size of the tricuspid orifice
• CXR—enlarged RA
• Cardiac catheter—the gradient across the tricuspid valve is measured.

Management

Diuretics may be required.

Surgical management

Recent ESC guidance[1] provides algorithms for the management of valvular heart disorders. Valves can be either repaired or replaced. The majority of valve replacements are to the aortic valve followed by the mitral valve. A brief overview of the types of surgical procedure used is given here. While many valve replacements require a sternotomy approach and cardiopulmonary bypass (CPB) there are now some procedures such as thoracoscopically assisted mitral valve surgery that utilizes a more minimally invasive approach.

Surgery will be discussed in more detail in Chapter 9.

Percutaneous valvuloplasty

MS may be treated percutaneously. The procedure is performed in a catheter laboratory using a similar approach to angiography: the catheter is passed transvenously into the RA; the atrial septum is punctured; and a valvuloplasty balloon is then inflated in the mitral valve to open up the stenosis.

An Echo is performed after the procedure, and the patient is usually discharged the following day. The patient may be left with a small shunt between the left and right atria, but this does not usually cause any problems.

Mitral valve repair

The annulus, chordae tendineae, or leaflets may be repaired surgically. However, if a patient has developed AF, they probably require anticoagulants and, ∴, the benefits of repair over replacement are negated.

Percutaneous mitral valve repair

New techniques for repair such as MitraClip® have been developed. This is predominantly for symptomatic patients who are not suitable for traditional surgical methods. The procedure can be done under general or local anaesthetic with sedation. A catheter is inserted via the femoral vein and the passes from the RA to the LA via a trans-septal puncture. The area of the mitral valve failing to close is secured. The patient will require close CVS monitoring for approximately 24h post procedure. An Echo and CXR is performed. The patient may have an arterial line, central line, and urinary catheter *in situ* initially. They may be given antibiotics and anticoagulation.

Transcatheter aortic valve implantation (TAVI or TAVR)

This approach is currently recommended for those patients with symptomatic AS not suitable for surgery. The procedure may be performed under general or local anaesthetic with sedation. A number of approaches can be used such as mini thoracotomy (usually done under general anaesthetic) direct aortic approach or insertion of a catheter via the femoral artery. A stent is placed in opening of the aortic valve and the diseased valve is obliterated. The new valve on a stent is placed in position. It can be either self-expanding or deployed using balloon inflation. The two types currently used are the balloon expandable Edwards-SAPIEN valve or the self-expanding Medtronic CoreValve.

The patient has rapid RV pacing during the operation and may continue to be paced post procedure. They will usually also have a urinary catheter and arterial line post procedure. Complications include:

- Stroke
- Tamponade
- Bleeding
- Limb ischaemia
- Bradyarrhythmia
- Pericardial effusion
- Acute renal failure

[1] Vahanian A, Alfieri O, Andreotti F, et al. (2012) Guidelines on the management of valvular heart disease (version 2012) The Joint Task Force on the Management of Valvular Heart Disease of the European Society of Cardiology (ESC) and the European Association for Cardio-Thoracic Surgery (EACTS). European Heart Journal **33**, 2451–96.

Valve replacement

Mechanical, tissue, or homograft (human) valves may be used for prosthetic valve replacement. Mechanical valves require the patient to take lifelong anticoagulant therapy. ∴, the choice of valve will be influenced by this factor. Other factors that may influence the choice are age, valve size, the valve to be replaced (>80% of mitral valve replacements are performed using mechanical valves because of the greater pressure difference across the closed mitral valve), availability (homografts), and clinical symptoms.

Mechanical valves

Mechanical valves have a long life expectancy. Anticoagulants will be given to prevent thrombus formation. The patient's international normalized ratio (INR) of prothrombin time should be checked regularly to ensure the correct dose of anticoagulant (usually warfarin) is given. The INR is kept higher in patients who have had a mitral valve, rather than aortic valve, replacement, because of the ↑ pressure on the mitral valve and ↑ turbulence in blood flow.

Mechanical valves may be tilting disk (Bjork–Shiley) or bi-leaflet (St Jude Medical—which is the most widely used type) in design (Fig. 4.1). These valves will click and this may be audible to the patient and their family. It is important that they are made aware of this and that it is normal.

Bioprosthetic valves (tissue valves)

Bioprosthetic valves may be porcine or pericardial in origin. Although they do not last as long as mechanical valves (~10–15yrs compared to >30yrs), the patient does not need to take anticoagulants and, ∴, they may be used in older patients or ♀ of child-bearing age.

Homografts

These are human valves. They are usually used for aortic valve replacements and are kept in valve banks around the country until required.

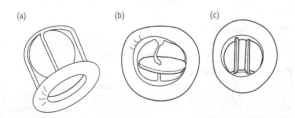

Fig. 4.1 Types of mechanical valves. (a) Ball and cage. (b) Tilting disc. (c) Bileaflet. Adapted with permission from Chikwe J, Beddow E, and Glenville B (2006). *Cardiothoracic Surgery*. Oxford University Press, Oxford.

Nursing considerations

The care of patients requiring heart-valve surgery will be discussed in Chapter 9. Points to remember are that patients may be young, may require valve replacement and CABG, and may require further valve surgery in the future. However, patients with valve problems may require admission to hospital for control of symptoms or tests related to their condition. Many of the symptoms experienced are related to either failure of the LV and, in some cases, right-sided heart failure. ∴, the treatment and nursing care will be similar to that discussed in Chapter 10.

Patients who have been diagnosed with heart-valve defects may not exhibit any symptoms for many years. ∴, they will need to be encouraged to report any development of symptoms, such as shortness of breath, palpitations, dizziness, and angina, because these may indicate that the defect is becoming worse. Some of the symptoms experienced may be confused with other disease processes or old age. All patients will need to attend regular out-patient follow-up, which may be every 6–12 months and will usually involve an Echo, ECG, and CXR. The development of new heart murmurs or conduction problems may be picked up at these appointments and again may indicate that the patient's condition has worsened. In some cases, murmurs may be severe enough to be heard by either the patient or their family.

Patients will need reassurance and guidance in relation to activities and exercise. For example, those patients with severe AS should avoid exercise because this may lead to arrhythmias and sudden death. Shortness of breath can be particularly frightening, especially when it happens at night. The nurse needs to advise the patient of ways to relieve this, such as lowering the legs over the side of the bed and supporting themselves in bed with more pillows. Weight gain also needs to be monitored because this can indicate that heart failure is progressing. As explained previously, it may be many years (if ever, in MVP) between diagnosis and symptom development, so where possible, patients need to be encouraged to carry on living a normal life.

If the heart-valve defect is the result of a genetic condition, such as Marfan's syndrome, genetic counselling for the patient and family will be required.

Driving restrictions

Patients with heart-valve problems are not able to hold a passenger-carrying vehicle/large goods vehicle licence while symptomatic.

Prevention of endocarditis

Endocarditis is discussed in more detail in Chapter 5. Guidance on endocarditis has changed. NICE[2] guidance suggests that antibiotic prophylaxis prior to dental and some other invasive procedures is no longer required for those at risk. However ESC[3] guidance suggests that it should be given to those at high risk undergoing highest risk dental procedures. Practices may ∴ vary as to who receives antibiotic prophylaxis which may cause some anxiety to the patient. Nurses need to be aware of the signs and symptoms of endocarditis so that they can assess their patients for these and also educate them regarding the importance of prevention. Patients should also be encouraged to have regular dental check-ups to help prevent endocarditis.

Anticoagulation

Patients who develop AF or have a mechanical valve replacement will be required to take an anticoagulant, usually warfarin. For mechanical valve replacement, anticoagulants need to be taken for life. Patients, ∴, will need educating regarding the side effects of warfarin, such as:

- Bleeding gums
- Bruising
- Blood in urine or stools
- Slower clotting time after any cuts or scrapes
- Interaction of warfarin with other medication (e.g. aspirin, some antibiotics, and some antiarrhythmics)
- Importance of not drinking alcohol to excess or binge drinking.

To establish the right dosage of warfarin, the patient will need to have regular blood checks to establish the INR. This should be done more frequently when the patient is first on the medication, to stabilize it. The INR is usually kept at 2.5 for patients with AF. The INR is kept higher for MVR compared with AVR, because the mitral valve is subject to more turbulent blood flow.

[2] National Institute for Health and Clinical Excellence (2008) *Prophylaxis Against Infective Endocarditis*. NICE, London.

[3] European Society Taskforce (2009) Guidelines on prevention, diagnosis and treatment of infective endocarditis. European Heart Journal **30**, 2369–413.

Related guidance

National Institute for Health and Clinical Excellence (2007) *Thoracoscopically Assisted Mitral Valve Surgery*. NICE, London

National Institute for Health and Clinical Excellence (2009) *Percutaneous Mitral Valve Leaflet Repair for Mitral Regurgitation*. NICE, London

National Institute for Health and Clinical Excellence (2010) *Percutaneous Mitral Valve Annuloplasty*. NICE, London.

National Institute for Health and Clinical Excellence (2012) *Transcatheter Aortic Valve Implantation for Aortic Stenosis*. NICE, London

Vahanian A, Alfieri O, Andreotti F, *et al.* (2012) Guidelines on the management of valvular heart disease (version 2012) The Joint Task Force on the Management of Valvular Heart Disease of the European Society of Cardiology (ESC) and the European Association for Cardio-Thoracic Surgery (EACTS) *European Heart Journal* **33**, 2451–96.

Chapter 5

Infective endocarditis

Introduction

Infective endocarditis (IE) is a condition that most commonly occurs in patients with pre-existing valve disease. Nurses working in the cardiac arena should be aware of those patients who are at risk of developing IE and its clinical management. This chapter covers the aetiology, diagnosis, treatment, nursing considerations, and specific educational issues that are relevant to the overall management and prevention of IE.

Aetiology

IE occurs when the endocardium is exposed to an infecting organism, with resultant colonization and tissue damage. It occurs mainly in susceptible hosts and a 1° component of this susceptibility is a roughened endocardial surface. It most commonly occurs in people with pre-existing cardiac lesions, although these may be minor and may not have resulted in haemodynamic problems. Vegetations develop when fibrin, platelets, and white cells adhere to the uneven surface and, consequently, micro-organisms carried in the bloodstream attach to them and multiply. In time, the vegetations can calcify. Vegetations tend to occur on regurgitant rather than stenotic valves and are usually present on the low-pressure side of the valve (i.e. the atrial side of the mitral valve and the ventricular side of the aortic valve). The vegetations tend to be large and friable and can project from the valve cusps, though they may be small and difficult to diagnose. If left untreated, this can result in valvular incompetence, regurgitation, subvalvular abscess, infective emboli, and rupture of supporting structures. Left-sided IE is much more common than right-sided IE; the most commonly affected valve is the mitral valve. Right-sided IE is commonly related to IV drug use and mostly affects the tricuspid valve. Right-sided endocarditis tends to be more benign and responds better to treatment. However, the sequelae of IE can be catastrophic in terms of cardiac function, sepsis, and embolic events. If left untreated, IE will invariably result in death.

Types of endocarditis

IE has been classified as follows:[1]

IE according to localization of infection and presence or absence of intracardiac material

- Left-sided native valve endocarditis (NVE). NVE has ↓ mortality than prosthetic valve endocarditis (PVE), but both are considered to be life threatening. NVE can occur on a previously normal valve, but this is rare.
- Left-sided PVE. This is divided into early- and late-onset PVE. Early-onset PVE occurs <1yr of prosthetic valve implantation and is usually caused by contamination of the valve at the time of implantation or from IV lines or urinary catheters. Late-onset PVE occurs >1yr after prosthetic valve implantation and is more likely to result from an infective organism that generally causes NVE.
- Right-sided IE.
- Device-related IE (PPM or ICD).

IE according to the mode of acquisition

- Healthcare associated IE: nosocomial (IE developing in a patient >48h after admission) or non-nosocomial (IE <48h after admission)
- Community-acquired IE
- IV drug abuse-associated IE.

Active IE

- E.g. fever, + blood cultures, evidence of IE.

Recurrence

- Relapse: repeat episodes caused by same microorganism <6mths after initial episode
- Reinfection: either different organism or the same organism but >6mths after the initial episode

---

[1] The Task Force on the Prevention, Diagnosis and Treatment of Infective Endocarditis of the European Society of Cardiology (ESC) (2009) Guidelines on the prevention, diagnosis, and treatment of infective endocarditis (new version 2009). *European Heart Journal* **30**, 2369–413.

Predisposing factors

There are several factors that can predispose individuals to developing IE:
- Prosthetic valves—the subvalvular ring is a common site in mechanical valves.
- Congenital heart disorders—mostly those with high-flow or turbulent jet streams (e.g. tetralogy of Fallot, VSD, bicuspid aortic valve, PDA, and coarctation of the aorta).
- Valvular heart disease—most commonly AR, AS, and MR.
- History of rheumatic fever, because this can damage cardiac valves. The incidence of rheumatic fever is now ↓ because of the use of antibiotics; however, many older patients may have had rheumatic fever in childhood.
- Gender—♂ are at higher risk of IE than ♀, although the reasons for this are not fully understood.
- Recurrent bacteraemia—this is common in IV drug users and those with severe periodontal disease or colon cancer. IE associated with body piercing and/or tattooing is an ↑ consideration.
- Invasive procedures in any individual who has other predisposing factors—e.g. dental, gynaecological, urological, or gastrointestinal surgery.
- Device related—IE can develop on pacemaker or ICD wires with or without associated valve involvement.

Common infective organisms

- *Streptococcus viridans*. Common after dental work and the most frequent causative organism in NVE.
- *Streptococcus bovis*. This is common in patients with underlying colon cancer.
- *Enterococcus faecalis*. Common in elderly ♂ after genitourinary surgery and in young ♀ after gynaecological procedures and childbirth.
- *Staphylococcus aureus*. Common in NVE and IV drug users. It often causes metastatic abscesses.
- *Staphylococcus epidermidis*. The most common cause of PVE.
- Fungi, such as *Candida albicans* and *Aspergillus* spp., cause PVE less commonly.

Signs and symptoms

Patients may present with acute symptoms, such as rigors and heart failure, when the causative organism is particularly virulent, but in the majority of patients the onset is insidious and malaise and pyrexia are common complaints. Patients often ignore symptoms, believing them to be influenza; however, fever is the most frequent sign of IE occurring in ~90% of patients. In patients at risk of developing IE, it is important to make a full assessment when influenza-like symptoms occur because these could be early symptoms. If these early symptoms are not treated, the patient will present with a characteristic clinical picture that includes the following:

- Heart murmur—usually a new murmur or a change in character of an existing murmur. This is usually caused by valve destruction.
- Pyrexia—may be low grade.
- Petechiae—these may develop on any part of the body (e.g. Roth's spots [retina] and Janeway lesions [palms and soles of feet]).
- Splinter haemorrhages in the nail beds.
- Osler's nodes—tender nodules on the tips of fingers and toes.
- Microscopic haematuria.
- Neurological problems, such as embolic occlusion of cerebral vessels or cerebral abscess.
- Cardiac problems, such as heart failure, palpitations, tachycardia, atrioventricular (AV) block—these are usually later manifestations, following destruction of valves and supporting structures.

Diagnosis

Because symptoms are often nonspecific, it can be difficult to make a definitive diagnosis. IE is usually suspected on the basis of clinical presentation and predisposing factors. TTE should be performed. If this is negative but IE is strongly suspected then TOE is indicated. Most clinicians use the Duke criteria to facilitate diagnosis. This involves identifying major and minor criteria: a definitive diagnosis can be made in the presence of two major criteria, one major criterion and three minor criteria, or five minor criteria.

Major criteria

- Positive blood cultures—persistently positive blood cultures over a 12h period with a typical microorganism for IE.
- Evidence of endocardial involvement— vegetation, abscess, or dehiscence of a prosthetic valve seen on echocardiography.
- Single positive blood culture for *Coxiella burnetii* or phase 1 IgG antibody titre >1:800.

Minor criteria

- Pyrexial >38°C
- Known predisposition to endocarditis
- Vascular phenomena (e.g. arterial emboli)
- Immune phenomena (e.g. Roth's spots)
- Microbiological evidence

Other investigations

- Bloods—full blood count (FBC), urea and electrolytes (U&E), liver function test (LFT), erythrocyte sedimentation rate (ESR), C-reactive protein (CRP)
- ECG—conduction defects may be present
- CXR
- Dental X-ray
- Urinalysis
- Immunology.

Clinical management

Management of the patient diagnosed with IE depends on their presenting symptoms, but the first-line treatment for all cases of IE is IV antibiotics. The antibiotics selected will depend on the causative organism isolated. Three sets of blood cultures are usually performed prior to IV antibiotics being commenced. Appropriate antibiotics are usually prescribed following advice from a microbiologist—combination therapy has been shown to be more effective than a single agent. Combinations of benzylpenicillin and gentamicin are commonly used to treat streptococcal infections and flucloxacillin and gentamicin and/or rifampin for staphylococcal infections. Vancomycin is used for those patients with penicillin allergies. Antifungals will be given to IE caused by fungi. The duration of treatment is usually several weeks (normally 2–6wks for NVE and at least 6wks for PVE) and, ∴, it is preferable to use a central line for their administration. A tunnelled central line further ↓ the probability of the catheter itself becoming infected.

The patient will also be symptomatically treated (e.g. with antipyretics to ↓ fever). They will also require ongoing monitoring and are likely to have serial echocardiography, ECG, and blood cultures.

Surgical intervention, such as valve replacement surgery, may be necessary, but, in most cases, medical management to control the infection is required before this. Surgery during the active phase carries ↑ risk.

Surgery is indicated for the following reasons:
• Developing heart failure
• Persistent infection despite antibiotic therapy
• Prevention of embolization (↑ risk with large, mobile vegetations)
• PVE (cure with antibiotics alone is unlikely).

Nursing considerations

The nursing management of patients with IE is dependent upon their symptoms. The main principles of nursing care are to:
- Administer antibiotics and evaluate their effectiveness.
- Manage symptoms, such as fever or night sweats.
- Monitor cardiovascular status and observe for potential complications.
- Support the patient's psychological needs.

The following are considered essential for all patients with a diagnosis of IE (frequency of observations may be reduced as their condition improves):
- Record temperature at least every 4h—↑ frequency if rigors occur, if the patient feels feverish or if temperature ↑. When the patient begins to feel better, they may wish to record their own temperature so appropriate teaching will be required.
- Monitor BP and HR to assess cardiovascular status at least every 4h—↑ frequency if symptoms deteriorate.
- Monitor respiratory rate and oxygen saturation (SaO₂) at least every 4h. Administer supplemental O₂ as prescribed.
- Monitor for evidence of neurological events (e.g. stroke, TIA). These will develop in 20–40% of patients with IE.
- Daily monitoring to detect embolic events: urinalysis for blood, observing skin for petechiae and nail beds for splinter haemorrhages.
- Daily 12-lead ECG: note any evolving AV blocks, e.g. prolonged P–R intervals.
- Observe IV site for signs of inflammation or infection whenever administering antibiotics. Change dressings as required. Peripheral cannulae will require resiting every 72h (check local policy).
- If the patient is relatively immobile, it is wise to measure and fit antiembolism stockings.
- Assessment of the risk of developing pressure ulcers is also indicated because patients presenting with IE may be anorexic, malnourished, and immobile. Preventative measures will need to be implemented depending on the risk assessment score.
- Nutritional assessment is imperative—many patients presenting with IE are anorexic and may have experienced weight loss. Referral for dietary supplements may be necessary.
- Antibiotic therapy will probably last for 4–6wks and a prolonged hospital stay is usually required. This may lead to depression, anxiety, and loss of self-esteem. It is, ∴, important to engage the patient and their family in discussions about their care and treatment. Information about probable length of stay and expected outcomes are essential in helping the family to cope with the situation. The patient may require financial support and referral to a social worker may be necessary.

Patient education

Because a previous episode of IE is a predisposing factor for further episodes, it is vital that the patient is aware of this. They need to know about
potential symptoms that should not be ignored and warrant further investigation and also the precautions they need to take to ↓ risk of future
infection. The patient will receive regular follow-up and monitoring of
their condition following discharge and it is important that they are aware
of this and attend all necessary appointments. Some patients may be sent
home with a temperature chart so may require teaching in accurately
recording their temperature.

Preventive measures largely consist of ↓ risk of bacterial contamination
from invasive procedures. ✐ Antibiotic prophylaxis is a controversial issue
as some guidance[2] suggests antibiotic prophylaxis for those at highest risk
undergoing high-risk procedures whereas NICE guidance[3] suggests that
antibiotic prophylaxis is not required.

High-risk patients are considered to be those with prosthetic valves,
previous history of IE, and some congenital heart defects. High-risk procedures are considered to be some dental procedures such as tooth extraction, root canal treatment, and scaling.

Individual clinicians may choose to prescribe antibiotics and further
research is being carried out in this area.

However, the need for regular dental check-ups and good oral hygiene
cannot be overemphasized in those at risk. For women of child-bearing
age who are at risk, it is advisable to avoid using intrauterine contraceptive devices.

A special note is required for IV drug users who are being discharged,
because the risk of recurrence is high in this group of patients. Referral
for rehabilitation to combat their addiction is recommended, but this will
only work on a voluntary basis. If the patient is not willing to be referred,
it is crucial that they are taught about the principles of asepsis and the
importance of skin cleansing and using clean needles in an attempt to ↓
their risk of reinfection.

---

[2] The Task Force on the Prevention, Diagnosis and Treatment of Infective Endocarditis of the
European Society of Cardiology (ESC) (2009) Guidelines on the prevention, diagnosis, and treatment of infective endocarditis (new version 2009). *European Heart Journal* **30**, 2369–413.

[3] National Institute for Health and Clinical Excellence (2008) *Prophylaxis Against Infective
Endocarditis*. NICE, London. ✐ http://www.nice.org.uk

Related guidance

National Institute for Health and Clinical Excellence (2008) *Prophylaxis Against Infective Endocarditis*. NICE, London

The Task Force on the Prevention, Diagnosis and Treatment of Infective Endocarditis of the European Society of Cardiology (ESC) (2009) Guidelines on the prevention, diagnosis, and treatment of infective endocarditis (new version 2009). *European Heart Journal* **30**, 2369–413.

Chapter 6

Coronary heart disease: stable angina

Introduction

CHD remains one of the largest causes of premature death in the UK.[1]
Angina is the most common symptom of CHD. It is usually described as
a central, retrosternal pain or ache that is crushing or choking in nature.
Pain may radiate down the left arm and/or up into the neck and is often
accompanied by shortness of breath (SOB) and sweating. Some patients
may describe it as chest discomfort. The presentation of CHD, however,
covers a broad spectrum of clinical signs and symptoms that vary in
severity. An individual may be asymptomatic despite disease within the
coronary arteries; may present with gradually worsening symptoms of
angina; or the first presentation may be death following an acute MI.

The progress of the disease is variable, depending on the individual's risk
factors and the coronary arteries affected. Terminology varies but, generally speaking, CHD is divided into two subtypes:

- Stable angina—with reversible ischaemia.
- Acute coronary syndromes (ACS)—which is an umbrella term that
  includes unstable angina and MI.

This chapter outlines the pathophysiology and clinical management of stable angina and Chapter 7 focuses on ACS.

Pathophysiology

Atherosclerosis

CHD is caused by atherosclerosis within the coronary arteries (commonly known as 'hardening of the arteries'). It is a progressive disease which is not thought to be part of the normal ageing process, but is associated with an interaction between endothelial injury, the inflammatory response, and dietary and blood lipids. Several theories attempt to explain the atherosclerotic process in arteries, but there is some debate about which is the most important factor. The following events are generally accepted to occur:

- Endothelial activation or damage stimulates the release of inflammatory mediators. The chemicals in tobacco and an ↑ low-density lipoprotein (LDL) level might be two of the common initiators of this response. It is also postulated that turbulent blood flow associated with ↑ BP might also result in endothelial damage.
- Inflammatory mediators recruit monocytes and lymphocytes which cross the endothelium and accumulate in the intima, and also ↑ proliferation of smooth muscle cells.
- Monocytes mature into macrophages which consume LDL and eventually become lipid-laden foam cells that lose the ability to re-enter the circulation.
- Foam cells, ∴, accumulate in the subendothelial space where they coalesce, forming the fatty streaks of early atherosclerosis. Fatty streaks may be present in the arteries of children affected by CHD, but they do not impede blood flow or ↓ the lumen size of the artery. Consequently, they are unlikely to produce symptoms of CHD but may be the precursors of more malignant atherosclerotic plaques.
- As the disease progresses, fibrogenic mediators are released in an attempt to remodel the fatty streaks, resulting in the replication of smooth muscle cells. These cells, and associated deposition of connective tissue, forms atherosclerotic plaques.
- Plaques initially cause outward remodelling of the artery, but eventually impinge on the lumen of the artery, restricting the flow of blood through it. This results in the progressive ↓ of available O_2 to the myocardium, which is especially marked when myocardial O_2 demand ↑ and the symptoms of stable angina are a direct consequence of this.
- The damage to the endothelium results in an inability of the vessel to control blood flow by local vasoconstriction or vasodilatation.
- Advanced plaques, which have a fibrous coating and a lipid-rich core, are unstable and liable to rupture or ulcerate. Consequently, thrombi form on the plaque surface, which ultimately further restricts the lumen of the artery and produces the symptoms of ACS (☐ Identifying patients with acute coronary syndromes (ACS), p.122).

Other causes

Myocardial ischaemia and the symptoms of angina can be produced by causes other than atherosclerosis, e.g. anaemia. Other common causes are coronary artery spasm and syndrome X, both of which will be briefly discussed here.

Coronary artery spasm

Vasospasm of a coronary artery can cause partial or complete obstruction of the vessel, resulting in myocardial ischaemia and angina. This often occurs at rest and is usually referred to as variant or Prinzmetal angina. The cause of vasospasm is unknown in most cases, but it can occur in arteries with or without atherosclerotic changes. ↑ in coronary vasomotor tone or spasm can result in acute MI or mimic STEMI (persistent ST-segment elevation, ± biochemical cardiac marker release). Nitrates and calcium-channel blockers are usually used to manage coronary artery spasm (🕮 Nitrates, p.369; Calcium-channel blockers, p.368).

Syndrome X

Patients with syndrome X present as follows:
- History of angina.
- Positive ETT.
- No evidence of coronary vasospasm.
- Normal coronary arteries on angiography.
- Myocardial contractility abnormalities are sometimes evident.
- Extreme fatigue.

Syndrome X is more common in ♀ than ♂, particularly ♀ who are commencing or have been through the menopause: oestrogen deficiency and other endocrine and metabolic factors are thought to be implicated. Prognosis for syndrome X is good. Treatment depends on the probable cause but can take the form of normal antianginal or oestrogen therapy. Relaxation techniques can be useful.

Clinical management

Principles of nursing management

Patients who present with stable angina are not usually admitted to hospital, unless ACS are suspected. In some cases, the symptoms of angina are only picked up in routine screening or health assessment. It is, ∴, imperative that the nurse undertakes a thorough cardiac assessment. Patients may be seen by a nurse in a rapid access chest pain clinic. Recent NICE guidance[1,2] has suggested a pathway for those presenting with chest pain (Fig. 6.1) and a management pathway for those diagnosed with stable angina (Fig. 6.2). The principles of nursing management with the patient presenting with angina are as follows:

* Assessment for symptoms—such as SOB, chest discomfort, fatigue, and palpitations. Assessment should include precipitating factors, location and duration of chest discomfort or pain, symptom severity, and a description of symptoms (🕮 General assessment of the patient, p.27).
* It is important to ascertain if symptoms are cardiac in origin. (🕮 Differential diagnosis of chest pain, p.30). In some patients, the presentation of angina might be confused with symptoms of other conditions (e.g. indigestion).
* Vital signs—temperature, pulse, BP, respiratory rate, and SaO_2.
* 12-lead ECG—may be normal but this does not rule out angina. If the patient is experiencing pain, ST-segment depression or T-wave abnormalities may be noted. Patients presenting with coronary vasospasm may have transient ST-segment elevation.
* Assessment of risk factors (🕮 Risk factors for cardiovascular disease, p.9).

Further nursing management includes:

* Lifestyle modification (🕮 Modifiable risk factors: 1, p.12—including referral to other services (e.g. a cardiac-rehabilitation nurse).
* Reassurance—anxiety can exacerbate symptoms; ∴, reassurance is crucial.
* Advice—include an explanation of the condition and any investigations that the patient may require.
* Symptom management—angina can be precipitated by strong emotions, exercise, cold weather, or eating a heavy meal and, ∴, patients should be advised accordingly. Also advise patients of the symptoms of a heart attack, and the need to seek help urgently if they occur.

[1] National Institute for Health and Clinical Excellence (2010) *Chest Pain of Recent Onset.* NICE, London.

[2] National Institute for Health and Clinical Excellence (2011) *Management of Stable Angina.* NICE, London.

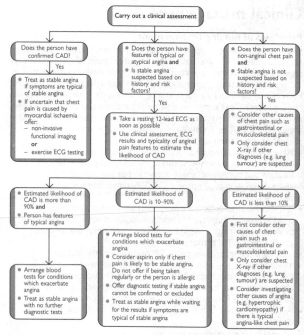

Fig. 6.1 Pathway for people presenting with stable chest pain. Adapted with permission from National Institute for Health and Clinical Excellence (2010) *Chest Pain of Recent Onset.* NICE CG95.

Investigations

Investigations may be performed after hospital admission or on an out-patient basis. The role of the nurse is to ensure that the patient understands why the investigations are necessary, what is involved, and what the consequences of the results may be. The type of investigations the patient will require should be determined by their estimated likelihood of CAD (NICE[3]). Chapter 3 provides a more detailed explanation of some of these investigations. Recommended investigations may include:

- Imaging studies: computed tomography calcium scoring (🕮 p.78)
- Myocardial perfusion scintigraphy (🕮 p.76)
- Stress Echo (🕮 Echocardiography, p.74)
- MRI (🕮 Cardiac magnetic resonance (CMR) imaging, p.77)
- ETT
- Coronary angiography (🕮 Coronary angiography: preprocedure care, p.139)
- Blood test including determination of troponin, serum glucose, serum cholesterol, a FBC, and serum U&E.

[3] National Institute for Health and Clinical Excellence (2010) *Chest Pain of Recent Onset*. NICE, London.

Medical management

Medical treatment aims to control symptoms and ↓ the risk of ACS or sudden cardiac death occurring. These factors, ∴, influence the management of the patient with stable angina. The pathway for the management of stable angina can be seen in Fig. 6.2. All patients receive medication (Chapter 19), which normally includes a combination of antianginal drugs and also those for 2° prevention:

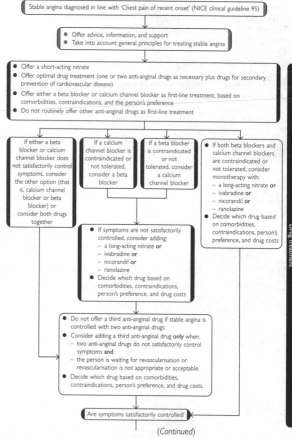

Fig. 6.2 Management of stable angina. Adapted with permission from National Institute for Health and Clinical Excellence (2011) *Management of Stable Angina*. NICE CG 126, NICE London.

(Continued)

- GTN (tablets or spray)—advise the patient to keep their medication with them at all times. Advise patients to use the medication before activities that normally induce their angina.
- β-blockers and/or calcium-channel blockers as first-line treatment.
- If these are ineffective or cannot be tolerated then other drugs may be added, e.g. long-acting nitrates or ivabradine or nicorandil or ranolazine.
- Aspirin.
- Statins.

Revascularization techniques, such as PCI or CABG, may be required. The need for this is usually assessed by coronary angiography.

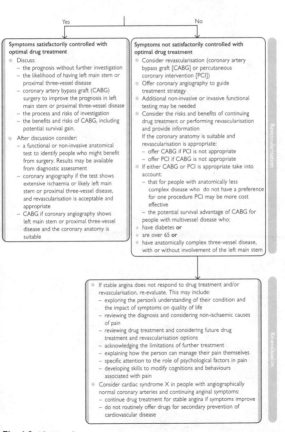

Fig. 6.2 (Continued)

Related guidance

National Institute for Health and Clinical Excellence (2010) *Chest Pain of Recent Onset.* NICE, London.

National Institute for Health and Clinical Excellence (2011) *Management of Stable Angina.* NICE, London.

Scottish Intercollegiate Guidelines Network (2007) *Management of Stable Angina.* SIGN, Edinburgh.

Acute coronary syndromes

Introduction

Despite a significant ↓ in mortality rates from CHD during the past four decades, statistics show that it continues to account for 80 000 deaths/yr in the UK, in contrast to 35 333 deaths/yr from lung cancer, 16 300 deaths/yr from colorectal cancer, and 12 141 deaths/yr from breast cancer.[1] Most deaths from CHD are a consequence of the 124 000 acute MIs which occur per year[1] and a significant proportion of these patients die before reaching hospital. CHD costs the NHS approximately £3.2 billion per year with hospital care accounting for 73% of the total cost.

The term ACS refers to a clinical spectrum of the same disease process, and includes unstable angina to non-ST-segment elevation MI (NSTEMI) and ST-segment elevation MI (STEMI). The common underlying cause results in the formation of a platelet-rich thrombus and reduced coronary arterial blood flow, which either partially or completely occludes the artery. When complete occlusion of a coronary artery occurs (STEMI) limitation of the infarct size is vital and thus rapid initiation of treatment is essential to obtain the greatest benefit. The development of services such as pre-hospital thrombolysis, direct delivery of patients from the ambulance to the catheter laboratory, and ↑ numbers of 24h 1° percutaneous coronary intervention (PPCI) facilities available have been important government initiatives that have been implemented to manage heart disease.

Central chest discomfort or pain remains the most common symptom that patients with an ACS report. Classically, the discomfort reported is retrosternal, radiating to the neck, jaw, and left shoulder or arm. In reality, symptoms are often ill-defined and the patient might describe a wide variety of symptoms that they do not initially associate with cardiac pain.

Treatment for this group of patients may be initiated and then continued across a variety of areas which include the pre-hospital/community setting, emergency department, coronary care unit, cardiac catheter laboratory, general ward, and chest pain unit. Nurses will encounter patients with both ST-segment elevation ACS and non-ST-segment elevation ACS at various points in their journey, thus clear and effective communication between healthcare providers across these different areas is imperative. With this in mind this chapter aims to outline the pathophysiology, methods for rapid diagnosis, and appropriate clinical management of ACS so that it that may be applied within any area and at any point in the patient's journey.

[1] British Heart Foundation Health Promotion Research Group (2010) *Coronary Heart Disease Statistics*. British Heart Foundation, London.

Pathophysiology

Rather than development and growth of an atherosclerotic plaque into a stenosis that limits blood flow, the symptoms and clinical conditions associated with ACS are, in general, related to the deterioration and rupture of an atherosclerotic plaque.

Certain factors ↓ the tensile strength of the plaque's fibrous cap, making it unstable or vulnerable. Pressure from the pulsating blood flow through the coronary artery creates either fissures through the endothelium down into the plaque or areas of endothelial desquamation, ↑ the plaque's vulnerability to sudden rupture/erosion and subsequent thrombus formation. The sudden rupture of an atherosclerotic plaque cap leads to the exposure of subendothelial collagen promoting platelet adhesion, activation, and aggregation, and a fibrin-rich thrombus develops. The presence of an occlusive or subocclusive thrombus overlying the plaque then results in ↓ coronary arterial blood supply. The pathological and clinical outcomes for patients who present with ACS depend on whether the thrombus partially or completely occludes the coronary artery, the degree of collateral blood supply to the myocardium, and the amount of myocardium affected.

- Complete coronary artery occlusion is responsible for *STEMI*—myocardial ischaemia leads to myocyte necrosis within 15–20min and spreads from subendocardium to subepicardium.
- Partial coronary artery occlusion is responsible for *non-ST-segment elevation ACS* and results in either unstable angina or NSTEMI.

In non-ST-segment elevation ACS, the formation of a thrombus is often associated with vasospasm, which causes intermittent obstruction to blood flow and fragments of the thrombus to break off and flow down the artery, where they lodge in smaller vessels. These distal emboli can therefore cause small areas of infarction without a complete occlusion of an epicardial vessel.

Identifying patients with acute coronary syndromes (ACS)

Because patients present with a wide variety of symptoms and with varying degrees of severity, the diagnosis of an ACS can be challenging. ACS should be suspected in those who describe any of the following symptoms:

- Severe central, crushing chest pain
- A heavy feeling, tightness, or a dull ache in the chest
- Discomfort in the chest, described as indigestion but associated with other symptoms of ACS
- A dull, numb, or tingling feeling in the chest or down the left arm.

Such pain/tightness/sensations might radiate to the any of the following parts of the body:

- Neck/jaw
- Down the left arm
- Down the right arm
- Across both shoulders
- Down both arms and into the fingers.

The following signs and symptoms may also be present, again in varying degrees of severity:

- Nausea
- Vomiting
- Sweating
- Pallor
- Cool and clammy peripheries
- Fear and anxiety.

Chest pain associated with ACS can occur at rest, be precipitated by exercise, or be associated with ↑ frequency and severity over a short period of time. For some it may be the worst pain they have ever experienced and for others much milder symptoms are mistaken for a non-cardiac cause to the extent that their presentation is significantly delayed. Other factors, e.g. stress, can be associated with an acute coronary event, and many patients, particularly ♀, also report recent fatigue and weakness before the event. A significant number of patients present with minimal symptoms or without any chest pain or discomfort at all. Such patients are more likely to be older, ♀, have hypertension, diabetes, and have a history of heart failure. Differential diagnosis of chest pain is discussed in Chapter 2 (📖 Differential diagnosis of chest pain, p.30).

Principles for immediate nursing care of all patients with suspected ACS

If ACS is suspected after the initial assessment of the patient's clinical signs and symptoms, the principles of nursing management are as follows:

- Manage patient in an area with a defibrillator and personnel skilled in resuscitation.
- 12-lead ECG—record an initial 12-lead ECG and repeat at regular intervals (i.e. every 10–15min) whilst symptoms are experienced. Record another 12-lead ECG when the patient is symptom-free and at intervals such as 60mins and 4h after symptoms have ceased.
- Vital signs—BP, pulse, respiratory rate, SpO_2, temperature—repeated, as the patient's condition dictates.
- Continuous cardiac monitoring.
- O_2 should only be administered if indicated by the SpO_2 levels. Optimum SpO_2 levels are >94% in patients without COPD and between 88–92% in those with COPD.
- Obtain venous access and take blood for determination of U&E, FBC, LFT, cholesterol levels, clotting time, glucose level, and cardiac markers. e.g. troponin T or I (according to local policy).
- Administer aspirin (300mg), as prescribed.
- Administer clopidogrel as prescribed.
- Administer S/L nitrate, e.g. GTN, as prescribed.
- Administer diamorphine or morphine by slow IV injection, as prescribed, and titrate to the patient's level of pain—aim for 1mg/min and observe the patient's level of consciousness and respiratory rate, particularly in elderly and frail patients.
- Ongoing assessment for symptoms—precipitating factors; location and duration of chest discomfort or pain; severity; description of symptoms (Ⅲ Chest pain, p.28).
- Reassurance—anxiety can exacerbate symptoms and, ∴, information provision and reassurance are vital.

Implementing appropriate treatment regimens is initially guided by the patient's symptoms and 12-lead ECG: treatment must not be delayed to await biochemical markers. The overall aim is common to all patients with ACS: relieve symptoms, resuscitate if needed, and prompt and effective restoration or preservation of coronary blood flow to relieve ischaemia and prevent further myocardial damage.

Patients with a *suspected* ACS must also be admitted to hospital for further assessment and potential treatment.

Specific principles for nursing patients with ST-segment elevation ACS: reperfusion

Patients with a good clinical history of ACS and the following criteria on their 12-lead ECG should be treated as a STEMI and must be rapidly assessed for reperfusion therapy (see Fig. 7.1). Individual hospital protocols vary slightly and ∴ it is vital that you check your local protocol. It is likely to include the following:

- ST-segment elevation >1mm in two contiguous limb leads.
- ST-segment elevation >2mm in two contiguous chest leads.
- Presumed new LBBB.
- Isolated ST-segment depression V1–V4, indicating a potential posterior infarct. The use of posterior leads V7, V8, and V9 (Fig. 7.2) will show ST elevation in those with a posterior STEMI. These additional leads will help identify those who will benefit from rapid reperfusion therapy.

Refer to Fig. 7.3 for the changes seen in the evolution of a STEMI. Table 7.1 shows the anatomical relationship of the leads on a 12-lead ECG. Figs 7.4 and 7.5 show 12-lead ECG changes in inferior and anterior STEMI.

Every effort must be made to restore blood flow in an obstructed coronary artery as quickly as possible, to limit the size of the infarct and minimize complications, such as arrhythmias and pump failure. Blood flow can be restored:

- Mechanically by PPCI (📖 PCI: preprocedure and postprocedure care, p.155), or
- Pharmacologically by the administration of thrombolysis.

Regardless of the reperfusion strategy employed, the most important factor is to start treatment as early as possible. Extensive research has shown that the prognosis for patients following an MI is closely related to the length of time the coronary artery remains blocked; the longer the duration of the blockage, the higher the mortality and morbidity results.

Evidence suggests that PPCI is superior to thrombolytic therapy[2]; it is associated with early patency rates exceeding 90% and low rates of serious bleeding, recurrent ischaemia, and death. In contrast patency rates following thrombolytic therapy can be as low as 50%. Current guidelines recommend that the delivery of PPCI should occur within 90min after the first medical contact or within 60min of arrival at the hospital (door-to-balloon time) (Fig. 7.1).[3] It is argued that if PPCI is unachievable within these timeframes then thrombolysis is preferred. If thrombolysis is used, coronary angiography should be performed within 24h.

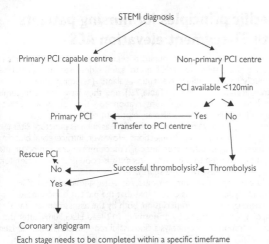

Fig. 7.1 STEMI reperfusion strategies. Information from Steg G, James SK, Atar D, Badano L, et al. (2012) ESC guidelines for the management of acute myocardial infarction in patients presenting with ST segment elevation. *European Heart Journal* **33**, 2569–619.

[2] DH (2008) *National Infarct Angioplasty Project (NIAP) Interim Report*. Department of Health & British Cardiovascular Society, London.

[3] Van de Werf F, Bax J, Betriu A, et al. (2008) Management of acute myocardial infarction in patients presenting with persistent ST-segment elevation. *European Heart Journal* **29**(23), 2909–945.

Specific principles for nursing patients with ST-segment elevation ACS

The role of the registered nurse in reperfusion therapy is effectively preparing the patient for PPCI or to safely administer the prescribed thrombolytics and adjunctive anticoagulants (assuming there are no contraindications to therapy (Table 7.2), and they have not been administered in another setting). Observation for the following potential post-STEMI complications is also an important role:

- Bleeding —usually limited to localized areas such as puncture sites (e.g. IV cannulas); avoid IM injections. However, intracerebral bleeding or bleeding from other sites, although much more rare, can occur and must be reported to the medical team (it is good practice to monitor the patient's Glasgow coma score).
- Failure to reperfuse from thrombolysis. After administration of a thrombolytic agent, it is crucial that that the patient is monitored for signs of successful reperfusion, both by the assessment of any ongoing symptoms and by performing a 12-lead ECG 90min after the administration of thrombolysis. Successful reperfusion is characterized by a >50% ↓ in the ST-segment 90min after the thrombolytic agent is administered. If the patient fails to reperfuse, they should be considered for rescue PCI.
- Acute LVF.
- Tachyarrhythmias (VT and VF).
- Reperfusion arrhythmias
- Transient or prolonged bradyarrhythmias—most commonly CHB (third-degree AV block) and Wenckebach's phenomenom (Möbitz type 1 second-degree AV block), which is usually associated with an inferior MI. These bradyarrhythmias can also occur in the presence of an anterior MI, although they are not usually transient and indicate an extensive infarct. (⎙ Atrioventricular blocks: second-degree heart block, p.218; Atrioventricular blocks: third-degree (complete) heart block, p.220) Möbitz II is more sinister. Accelerated idioventricular rhythm can also indicate reperfusion.
- Pericarditis (⎙ Pericardial disease, p.309).
- Cardiogenic shock (⎙ Cardiogenic shock, p.349).
- RV infarct associated with an inferior MI.
- Mitral valve regurgitation caused by papillary muscle dysfunction. (⎙ Mitral valve regurgitation, p.86)
- VSD.
- Procedural complications associated with PPCI (Table 8.1)

Table 7.1 Anatomical relationship of leads on the 12-lead ECG

Standard leads

- Septal wall – leads V1 and V2
- Anterior wall—leads V3 and V4
- Lateral wall—leads I, aVL, V5, and V6
- Inferior wall—leads II, III, and aVF

Nonstandard leads

- Right ventricle—right-sided chest leads V1 to V6R—most useful lead V4R (right ventricular MI has been reported in up to 50% of patients who present with an inferior MI, therefore a right-sided ECG is recommended)
- Posterior wall—leads V7 to V9

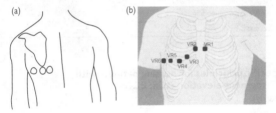

(a)

(b)

V7–posterior axillary line
V8–below the scapula
V9–paravertebral border

Each lead in the same horizontal plane
as V6

Fig. 7.2 (a) Lead position for a posterior ECG (b) Lead position for a right-sided ECG.

Table 7.2 Contraindications to thrombolysis

Absolute contraindications

- Active internal bleeding
- Recent head trauma and/or intracranial neoplasm
- History of cerebrovascular disease (haemorrhagic stroke at any time, ischaemic stroke within 1yr)
- Previous allergic reaction to streptokinase
- Recent (within last 2wks) surgery (including dental extraction)
- Aortic dissection

Relative contraindications

- Coagulation defects
- Known bleeding diatheses
- Severe uncontrolled hypertension
- Heavy vaginal bleeding
- Severe liver disease

Specific principles for nursing patients with ST-segment elevation ACS: ECGs
See Figs. 7.3, 7.4, 7.5.

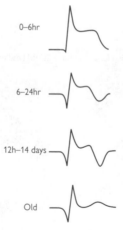

Fig. 7.3 Changes seen in the evolution of a ST-segment elevation MI.

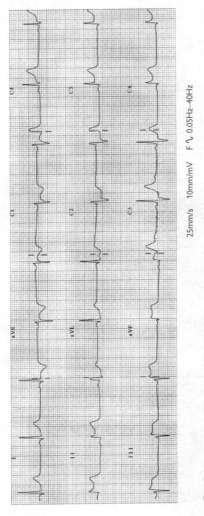

Fig. 7.4 Inferior lateral ST-segment elevation MI.

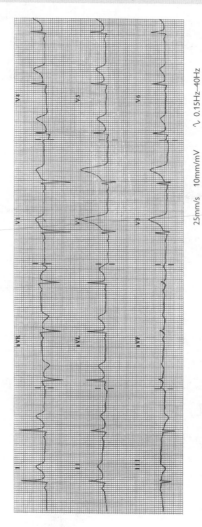

Fig. 7.5 Anterior ST-segment elevation MI.

Specific principles for nursing patients with non-ST-segment elevation ACS

In contrast to ST-segment elevation ACS, in which the risk of adverse events is highest in the first few hours, those with non-ST-segment elevation ACS are at highest risk following the event. It is on the basis of a characteristic pattern of release of cardiac markers (such as CK-MB, myoglobin, and troponin) which provides a diagnosis of a NSTEMI as opposed to unstable angina.

In addition to the principles of management outlined in 🕮 Principles for immediate nursing care of all patients with suspected ACS, p.123, the role of the registered nurse in the **ongoing** management of this group of patients also includes:

- Serial 12-lead ECG recordings, monitoring for abnormalities such as horizontal ST-segment depression or T-wave inversion.
- Measurement of cardiac markers on admission and 6–12h after symptom onset or according to local policy.
- Continuous monitoring of ongoing symptoms of ACS.
- Safe administration of medications—e.g. antiplatelet agents (aspirin and thienopyridines), antithrombin agents (low-molecular-weight heparin [LMWH], fondaparinux), β-blockers, ACE inhibitors, statins, and GP IIb/IIIa inhibitors.
- Risk stratifying patients and identifying those who might be at high risk of further adverse cardiac events.
- Highlight high-risk patients to the appropriate medical team.

Patients with the following features are at high risk of an adverse cardiac event:

- Horizontal ST-segment depression, which reverses when symptoms have resolved.
- Cardiac arrhythmias (bradyarrhythmias and tachyarrhythmias).
- Symptoms that continue regardless of analgesia, antiplatelet, and anticoagulant therapies.
- Haemodynamic instability.
- ↑ troponin I or T levels.
- Prolonged chest pain at rest (>20min) and recurrent pain at rest.
- Diabetes mellitus.
- Evidence of LVF.
- Aged >75yrs.
- Early postinfarction unstable angina.

Risk stratification of patients (i.e. identifying those who are at high or low risk of adverse events) with non-ST-segment elevation ACS helps to appropriately target both the type and the intensity of medical therapies and interventions. Several validated risk scores are available for use in clinical practice, however NICE (2010) recommend the Global Registry of Acute Coronary Events (GRACE) risk score.[4] The risk of 6mth mortality is calculated on the basis of clinical features at presentation including: age, heart rate, systolic BP, serum creatinine, Killip heart failure classification, cardiac arrest, ST-segment deviation, and biochemical markers. Without appropriate and rapid initiation of treatment patients with non-ST elevation ACS will remain at risk of further coronary events and sudden cardiac death. High-risk patients benefit from more aggressive treatment regimens, e.g. the administration of GP IIb/IIa inhibitor and angiography (with follow-on PCI if indicated) within 96h of first admission. Angiography will provide information on any underlying CHD so that the most suitable intervention (PCI, CABG, or medical management) can be identified and initiated. Those at low risk might be discharged early and safely from hospital.

4 National Institute for Health and Clinical Excellence (2010) *Unstable Angina and NSTEMI: The Early Management of Unstable Angina and Non-ST-Segment-Elevation Myocardial Infarction.* NICE, London. Clinical Guideline 94. ℘ http://www.nice.org.uk

Specific principles for nursing patients with ACS after initial acute presentation

This should include the following:

- Continuous cardiac monitoring—discontinuation of cardiac monitoring must be based on the individual patient's haemodynamic status. As a guide, patients should be free of pain and arrhythmias and haemodynamically stable for a minimum of 24h before discontinuation.
- Tight control of blood glucose levels in those with diabetes or a blood glucose level >11mmol/L on presentation.
- Monitor for signs of LVF (low SpO$_2$, tachycardia, SOB, ↑ respiratory rate)—particularly in patients with extensive anterior infarcts.
- Mobilizing patients after the acute phase must also be based on the patient's individual haemodynamic status after an acute cardiac event. Patients who recover without complications (i.e. those who are without cardiac arrhythmia or LVF and who are haemodynamically stable) can be mobilized from bed to chair within 12h of their acute event and gently mobilized using telemetry monitoring after 12–24h.
- Clear and timely provision of information regarding their condition. Advice and information provision regarding the aims of the patient's stay in hospital, an explanation of the condition, any investigations, and contact details for key organizations or individuals to contact on discharge should form the basis of the information provided.
- Assessment of risk factors (🕮 Risk factors for cardiovascular disease, p.9).
- Assessment of cardiac rehabilitation needs—might also require the patient to be referred to other services, e.g. cardiac rehabilitation nurse, dietician, or diabetic nurse (🕮 Cardiac rehabilitation, p.325).

Information on discharge must be individualized and should not be prescriptive. It should include the following:

- The causes of their condition.
- Risk factors for ACS and their management.
- Importance of physical activity (if able) and which activities are best—it is important to build up activity gradually on returning home, it is not safe to exercise when the patient has a viral infection.
- Exercise advice—regular moderate physical activity is best (unless the doctor advises against this) such as walking, cycling, swimming, dancing. Important to ↑ physical activity gradually, rest if feeling tired or breathless. Avoid activities after a large meal, or when the weather is very hot or cold.
- Appropriate and patient-specific dietary advice—including alcohol.
- Importance of relaxation.

Driving restrictions (up-to-date guidelines can be obtained from the DVLA website[5]).

- Return to work advice.
- When and how to use S/L nitrates.

- Information regarding all prescribed medications and their potential side effects—ensuring that the patient is clear when and how to take their medications.
- Advice on sexual activity—it is suggested that if an individual can climb a flight of stairs they should be able to safely participate in sexual activity. Some medications can interfere with sexual performance. The patient should discuss any worries or concerns with their doctor or nurse (📖 Sex, p.330).
- What follow-up to expect—such as GP clinics, 2° prevention clinics, cardiac rehabilitation programmes, local and national support groups, and out-patient appointments.
- Smoking cessation advice (if applicable) (📖 Smoking cessation, p.12) and community links.
- When to seek advice and help if symptoms recur (dial for an ambulance if chest pain >15min and not relieved by GTN).

Investigations

These are generally performed during hospital admission. The role of the nurse is to ensure that the patient understands the importance of the investigation, what it involves, and the potential consequences.

Potential investigations include:

- CT calcium scoring
- ETT
- Coronary angiogram
- Blood tests include biochemical cardiac markers, glucose, serum cholesterol, FBC, and U&E
- Echo
- CT angiogram (📖 Imaging studies: computed tomography calcium scoring, p.78).

Medical management

The aim of medical treatment is to control symptoms and reduce the risk of further acute coronary events or sudden cardiac death occurring. All patients will receive medications, see Chapter 19, which will generally include:

- GTN tablets or spray—the patient must be advised to keep this with them at all times
- Aspirin
- β-blocker
- Statin
- ACE-inhibitor
- Thienopyridine (e.g. clopidogrel).

Interventions

Interventions may include PCI.

---

5 🔗 http://www.dvla.gov.uk

Related guidance

Hamm CW, Bassand JP, Agewell S, et al. (2011) European Society of Cardiology Guidelines for the management of acute coronary syndromes in patients presenting without persistent ST segment elevation. *European Heart Journal* **32**, 2999–3054.

National Institute for Health and Clinical Excellence (2010) *Unstable Angina and NSTEMI*. Clinical Guideline 94. NICE, London.

National Institute for Health and Clinical Excellence (2011) *Hyperglycaemia in Acute Coronary Syndromes*. Clinical Guideline 130. NICE, London.

Steg G, James SK, Atar D, et al. (2012) ESC guidelines for the management of acute myocardial infarction in patients presenting with ST segment elevation. *European Heart Journal* **33**, 2569–619.

Thygesen K, Alpert J, Jaffe A, et al. (2012) Third universal definition of MI. *European Heart Journal* **33**, 2551–67.

Van de Werf F, Bax J, Betriu A, et al. (2008) Management of acute myocardial infarction in patients presenting with persistent ST-segment elevation. *European Heart Journal* **29**(23), 2909–45.

Wijns W, Kolh P, Danchin N, et al. (2010) ESC/EACTS guidelines on myocardial revascularisation. *European Heart Journal* **31**, 2501–55.

Related guidance

Chapter 8

Interventional cardiology for coronary heart disease

Introduction

CHD is by far the most common cause of heart disease, resulting from the narrowing of coronary arteries (stenosis). CHD accounts for 80 000 deaths per year in the UK.[1] Whether the cardiac nurse is working in CCU, an interventional unit, or a cardiothoracic surgical ward, they will at some stage be involved in caring for a patient who requires coronary angiography. This is a definitive test to diagnose the presence or absence of CAD, in addition to non-atherosclerotic causes of stable angina, such as coronary artery spasm.

If the diagnosis of CHD is made, the patient will be advised by the interprofessional team of the most suitable treatment option to meet their individual needs. This will be based on a number of factors including symptoms, the severity of the disease, and patient choice. The main treatment options available for the symptoms of CHD are:

• Conservative/medical management and modification of risk factors
• Revascularization by PCI or CABG.

It is essential to ensure patients are aware of the potential diagnostic outcomes and management options when they are being prepared for angiography. It is also important to reinforce the message that although treatment options offer an opportunity to alleviate symptoms, assist in 2° prevention and, in some cases, reduce the risk of death, there is no cure for CHD. CHD is an incurable and progressive disease.

The best treatment option for the patient depends on the extent and severity of their disease, the presence of any other diseases (comorbidity), and, of course, patient preference.

Surgical management and pharmacological options are discussed in Chapter 9 and Chapter 19. The purpose of this chapter is to give an overview of interventional cardiology. Diagnostic angiography and PCI are discussed, in addition to related issues (e.g. achieving haemostasis, pharmacological adjuncts, and complications). The principles of nursing care for both angiography and PCI are similar and will, ∴, be discussed together; any differences will be clarified.

Although coronary angiography is the focus of this chapter, it is worth noting that cardiac catheterization is the generic term which refers to a variety of procedures including angiography, ventriculography, and right or left heart catheterization. ∴ abnormalities of the heart valves, heart muscle and coronary arteries can be identified by these procedures.

[1] British Heart Foundation Health Promotion Research Group (2010). *Coronary Heart Disease Statistics*. British Heart Foundation, London.

Coronary angiography: preprocedure care

Coronary angiography (often referred to as 'cardiac catheterization') is the process whereby a radiopaque contrast medium is injected into the coronary circulation through a cardiac catheter under fluoroscopic X-ray. This provides anatomic and haemodynamic data that enables evaluation of the patency of coronary arteries and the heart's efficiency in circulating blood through the chambers.

Cardiac catheterization can be carried out through the arterial system (left heart catheter) or the venous system (right heart catheter), depending on the indication for the procedure and the information required.

To fully prepare and obtain the patient's consent and cooperation, it is essential to assess the patient's understanding and attitudes towards the procedure and address any misconceptions, including potential results and subsequent treatment. It is also useful to explain what to expect during the procedure:

- Cameras will move around throughout the procedure, sometimes close to the face, enabling the heart and arteries to be filmed from several different angles.
- The patient might experience a 'hot-flush' during one of the last pictures, because of the large volume of contrast medium injected. This could also cause the patient to feel as if they have voided urine, although this will not have happened.

Ensure informed patient consent is obtained, according to local policy, because this is a legal requirement.

Monitor and record a full set of baseline observations that include the following:

- HR and rhythm
- BP
- 12-lead ECG
- Respiratory rate
- Oxygen saturation (SpO_2)
- Temperature
- Weight and height
- Presence or absence of peripheral pulses (radial and pedal)
- Patients with diabetes mellitus require measurement of blood glucose.

Ensure all blood results are available if required:

- U&E and/or glomerular filtration rate (GFR)—if deranged, the patient may require prehydration and N-acetylcysteine (NAC)[2] to protect against contrast nephropathy.
- FBC and cross-match.
- A clotting screen if the patient usually takes warfarin.

Record administration and omission of medications, in particular the following:

- *Warfarin*—ensure the drug is discontinued 3 days before the procedure and that the INR is <1.7[2] to ↓ the risk of bleeding. Patients may require hospital admission for IV heparin therapy.

- *LMWH*—omit the dose on the morning of the procedure.
- *Patients with diabetes mellitus*—if the patient is fasting during a period in which diabetic medications are prescribed, these should be omitted. Patients should not take metformin on the morning of the procedure (risk of lactic acidosis). Ensure that all insulin-requiring patients with diabetes mellitus are prescribed sliding-scale insulin and IV fluids commencing on the morning of the procedure, to prevent risk of hypoglycaemic/hyperglycaemic episodes during the procedure. This is not required for tablet-controlled or diet-controlled patients; however, IV access is recommended. It is advisable to schedule patients with diabetes mellitus to have their procedure early in the day.
- *Clopidogrel & aspirin*—all patients undergoing an angiogram ± angioplasty should receive a stat dose of clopidogrel and aspirin, unless contraindicated or the patient is having planned cardiac surgery.

It is necessary for patients to fast, because the contrast medium can cause nausea and vomiting, or in severe disease, emergency surgery might be required. Patients should not receive food for up to 4h before the procedure. Clear fluids may be consumed up until the time of the procedure.[2]

The following practices are also recommended:
- To ↓ the risk of infection, the hair on the patient's arm or groin, depending on the site of access, should be *clipped* as close as possible to the time of procedure.
- Document any prostheses.
- Ensure venous access—the left arm is preferable because of the positioning of the equipment and personnel on the right side of the patient during the procedure.
- Document any allergies—including iodine/shellfish. Contrast medium contains iodine. Shellfish contains iodine and may indicate sensitivity to the contrast medium. If the patient has a known allergy, they might require prophylactic administration of hydrocortisone and antihistamine.
- If the patient has had a previous CABG, ensure that the operation notes are available.
- Ensure that the documentation/checklist is complete.
- If any observations/results are outside normal parameters, inform the operator.

---

[2] This may vary between institutions, so please refer to local policies.

Arterial access

There are three main arterial access sites for coronary angiography and intervention:

- The radial artery
- The femoral artery
- The brachial artery.

There are advantages and disadvantages for each route. A major advantage of both brachial and radial approaches is that they enable early mobilization post procedure, and in some cases, this is immediate. Access through the brachial artery often requires arterial cut-down and is, $\therefore$, technically more difficult and used infrequently.

Access through the femoral artery has several limitations, including prolonged bed rest post procedure, causing ↑ discomfort for the patient. It is also relatively contraindicated in patients with PVD or those requiring aggressive anticoagulation therapy. Patients with breathing difficulties or reduced LV function might not tolerate lying flat.

In practice, the radial and femoral arteries are used more frequently. The approach used should incorporate operator experience (because most operators are not proficient in gaining access through all three routes), patient preference, and the existence of comorbidities, such as PVD.

Coronary angiography: postprocedure care

The purpose of frequent patient observation after cardiac catheterization is to detect arterial or venous puncture-related complications, and systemic or disease-related events. Postprocedure care includes:

- A full set of observations—BP, HR, temperature, SpO_2, and respiratory rate.
- Colour, warmth, and sensation (CWS) of affected limb.
- Presence or absence of pedal/radial pulses (relevant to arterial access site).
- Wound site—observe for bleeding, haematoma formation, and signs of infection.

If the patient is unstable or complaining of chest pain:

- Attach patient to a cardiac monitor.
- Perform a 12-lead ECG and compare with preprocedure ECG findings to assess any detrimental changes/complications.
- Repeat full set of observations.
- Report to operator/nurse in charge.
- If necessary, give appropriate treatment (e.g. O_2, nitrate and analgesia).

The frequency of observations should be determined by the patient's condition; however, the following can be used as a guide for stable or routine patients:

- Monitor and record pulse and BP:
  - Every 30min for 2h
  - Every 1h until bed rest is complete
  - Include respiratory rate and SpO_2 if necessary.
- Monitor and record CWS of affected limb, pedal/radial pulse and wound site check:
  - Every 30min to 1h until bed rest is complete
  - 1h post mobilization
  - On the morning after the procedure and/or before discharge
  - Also refer to the sheath-removal section (Sheath removal, p.144).

The following are also important:

- Educate the patient to inform staff of any chest pain/breathlessness or bleeding/discomfort at the site of entry.
- Explain how to apply pressure to the femoral site if required (for coughing, sneezing, or if the patient feels any warmth or wetness in the area).
- Encourage the patient to drink oral fluids to flush the contrast medium from their system. The contrast medium could induce renal impairment.
- Patients should only be given a light diet until after sheath removal, because this might induce vomiting.

- Monitor urine output. If the patient fails to void urine within 6h of the procedure, or if the patient is in discomfort/has difficulty passing urine, a urinary catheter might be required.
- Emphasize the importance of bed rest, because moving or sitting up immediately postprocedure can induce bleeding or haematoma.

Bed rest following a femoral angiogram

Following haemostasis, the patient can lie at 45° for 1h. If no complications or signs of bleeding are observed, they can sit upright in bed. A total of 3h bed rest is recommended before mobilization.[3] If a haemostatic device is present, e.g. an AngioSeal™ (St Jude Medical, Stratford, UK), the amount of bed rest is ↓ (🕮 Achieving haemostasis: closure devices, p.147).

Bed rest following a brachial or radial angiogram

The radial arterial pressure device should be released slowly (🕮 Achieving haemostasis: closure devices, p.147). The patient should rest in a bed/chair for a total of 1–2h and avoid moving the affected arm. Following a brachial procedure, the sutures should be removed after 7 days, or after 10 days for patients with diabetes mellitus.

Patient education

Advise the patient of the following after angiography/before discharge:
- Report any bleeding or swelling at puncture site to a healthcare professional.
- Continue with prescribed medications.
- Avoid strenuous activity for 48h.
- Avoid a bath or shower for 24h.

Medication

- Metformin should be withheld for 48h postprocedure. If U&E were abnormal preprocedure, they should be rechecked (by GP if applicable) before recommencement.
- Recommence anticoagulant therapy on the evening of the procedure.

---

[3] This may vary between institutions, so please refer to local policies.

Sheath removal

Manual compression

Sheath removal is usually performed immediately after a diagnostic angiogram, unless heparin has been administered (e.g. during a prolonged or complicated angiogram) or the patient has received thrombolytic or glycoprotein GP IIb/IIIa therapy. If this is the case, or if an interventional procedure has taken place, then sheath removal generally occurs after a period of 3–6h.

The best approach for sheath removal is controversial, especially with the availability of new devices for closing femoral punctures (Achieving haemostasis: closure devices, p.147). This section will concentrate on manual compression.

Removing a sheath from an artery is not without risk and potential complications include the following:

• Bleeding at the site or retroperitoneal bleeding
• Pseudoaneurysm
• Arteriovenous fistula
• Distal ischaemia or necrosis
• Haematoma formation
• Arterial occlusion
• Vasovagal response, resulting in hypotension and bradycardia.

In an attempt to reduce the occurrence of complications, it is important to gather the following information before the procedure:

• *Has heparin been administered?* If so, it is important to determine the activated clotting time (ACT). This should usually be <150–165s. This figure varies between institutions, so refer to local standards.
• *What is the patient's BP?* If the patient is hypertensive (systolic BP >150mmHg), prolonged pressure will be required to achieve haemostasis. Antihypertensive medication might be required prior to sheath removal. If the patient is hypotensive, the cause should be treated.
• *Presence of a haematoma?* This can cause considerable discomfort to the patient and subsequently cause an ↑ in BP. Consider appropriate analgesia before sheath removal.
• *What is the patient's LV function?* This information can be obtained from the patient's medical notes. If the patient has ↓ LV function, greater caution/more frequent observation is required in the event of plasma substitute administration following a vasovagal reaction.

Preprocedure care

The procedure for femoral arterial sheath removal using manual compression is as follows:

• Explain the procedure and gain consent.
• Ensure the patient is free of chest pain.
• Perform observations, as described in the section on postprocedure care following angiography (Coronary angiography: postprocedure care, p.142).
• Ensure patent IV access.

- Gather the required equipment (Box 8.1) and prepare the trolley.
- Ensure the patient is lying flat (i.e. with one pillow).
- Connect the patient to a cardiac monitor and set the noninvasive BP cuff to check patient's BP every 3–5min. Again, practice varies considerably between institutions, and in some areas, this is only required following an interventional procedure.
- Ensure another nurse, who is accredited in IV drug administration, is nearby, in case of emergency. Also ensure that the nurse call bell is within reach.
- Ensure emergency medications, such as plasma substitute and atropine, are prescribed. If a prescription is required for the use of a Femostop® in the Trust in which you work, ensure this is written prior to sheath removal.

Box 8.1 Equipment required for femoral sheath removal
- Dressing trolley/tray
- Sterile dressing pack
- Sterile gauze swabs
- Sterile gloves
- Bioclusive dressing
- Sterile normal saline sachet (for cleansing)
- Protective goggles
- Protective apron
- Saline flush
- Femostop® equipment
- Atropine 600mcg
- Plasma substitute 500mL and blood-giving set.

Procedure
- Wash and dry hands.
- Put on protective clothing/equipment.
- Remove the bioclusive dressing and clean the area using an aseptic technique.
- Locate the femoral pulse by palpation of the femoral groin (~1–2cm above the puncture site). Place the index and middle fingers on the pulse and exert pressure while removing the sheath with the other hand. If a venous sheath was also inserted, it is advisable to remove the arterial sheath first and remove the venous sheath after ~10min. The venous sheath is innermost.
- Observe the patient for signs of complications—vasovagal response can induce bradycardia, hypotension, nausea, vomiting, yawning, sweating, pallor, and/or agitation.
- If necessary, call the second nurse to administer atropine and/or plasma substitute, as required.
- Apply continuous pressure for a minimum of 10min (diagnostic) or 15–20min (interventional). Release pressure slowly and continue to press lightly, as appropriate.

- While applying reduced pressure with one hand, palpate the surrounding area with the other hand, to detect haematoma formation. The skin should be soft and pliable.
- If bleeding persists or a haematoma is enlarging, apply further pressure and assess whether a compression device is required (📖 Achieving haemostasis: closure devices, p.147).
- When haemostasis is achieved, clean the area using sterile normal saline and apply a biocclusive dressing.
- Document the time of haemostasis.

Postprocedure care

Nursing care following sheath removal is the same as the postprocedure care following coronary angiography (📖 Coronary angiography: postprocedure care, p.142).

Achieving haemostasis: closure devices

Cardiac nurses often encounter patients following invasive diagnostic or interventional procedures. Following these procedures, introducer sheaths are removed. Haemostasis can be achieved using either manual digital compression or a vascular closure device. Achieving haemostasis of the femoral artery by manual compression requires physical strength and stamina for lengthy periods and can be uncomfortable for the patient and health professional. The majority of closure devices offer the advantages of early ambulation and patient comfort, with the exception of the Femostop® device.

A variety of closure devices are currently available, including bioabsorbable plug devices (AngioSeal™ [St Jude Medical, Stratford, UK], VasoSeal™ [Datascope, Cambridgeshire, UK] and ExoSeal™ [Cordis Corporation, New Jersey, USA]), percutaneous suture-closure devices (PerClose® [Abbott Vascular, Maidenhead, UK]) and external aids to manual compression (Femostop® and Radistop® [Radi Medical Systems, Surrey, UK] and the TR Band™ [Terumo Medical Corporation, Tokyo, Japan]). Other methods are also employed for vascular closure, including staple devices (StarClose™ [Abbott Vascular, Maidenhead, UK]) and surface patches.

The principles of care for a patient with a vascular closure device *in situ* are the same as those described in the postprocedure section (📖 Coronary angiography: postprocedure care, p.142). Frequent observation of the wound site needs to be maintained because the risk of complications is not eliminated by using a device. The use of closure devices varies between institutions; it is, ∴, important to determine which devices are used in your area. It is also important to seek guidance and training for optimal use of the device. The following is an overview that describes the main closure devices available:

AngioSeal™

This device creates a seal by sandwiching the puncture site between a bio-absorbable anchor and a collagen sponge. These dissolve in ~2–3mths.

VasoSeal™

This system delivers collagen extravascularly to the surface of the femoral artery. The collagen attracts and activates platelets in the arterial puncture, forming a clot and, ∴, resulting in a seal at the arterial puncture site.

ExoSeal™

The ExoSeal™is indicated for femoral artery puncture site closure following diagnostic or interventional catheterization procedures. This system delivers a biobasorbable polyglycolic acid (PGA) plug which is held in place by the femoral fascia outside the arteriotomy site. Haemostasis is therefore achieved without impeding arterial flow. The plug is absorbed within 60–90 days.

PerClose®

The PerClose® is a percutaneous suture-closure device that is not dependant on clot formation and can be used in anticoagulated patients.

StarClose™

The StarClose™ consists of a 'star'-shaped clip, which is designed to promote the 1° healing process to achieve closure of femoral access sites following both diagnostic and interventional procedures.

Femostop®

The Femostop® is a manual compression system, which consists of an arch with a pneumatic pressure dome, a belt and a reusable pump, with a manometer, for inflation. The pressure dome is placed over the vessel puncture site in the groin and the belt is placed around the patient. The dome applies a mechanical pressure over the vessel puncture site, inducing haemostasis.

Radistop®

Radistop® is a manual compression system for the radial artery. It consists of a support plate, a compression pad and a strap. The compression pad is placed over the puncture site and pressure is maintained using the velcro straps. The manufacturer recommends that pressure is maintained for 30–60min for a diagnostic procedure and 3–4h for an interventional procedure.

TR Band™

The TR Band™ is a transparent radial compression device indicated for radial artery puncture closure following diagnostic and interventional procedures. The TR Band provides controlled compression of the radial artery without occluding vessel flow or compressing local nerve structures. The transparent band enables visualization of the insertion point while the injection port and inflator syringe allows accurate pressure adjustment.

Complications of coronary angiography

Prevention and detection of complications are the main aims of nursing care, both during and after angiography. Although complications are rare, they do occur and can be life threatening; ∴, early detection and intervention are essential. It is important to recognize complications. The complications discussed here are associated with both angiography and PCI.

Peripheral vascular complications

- *Bleeding*—use manual pressure or a compression device to achieve haemostasis during sheath removal.
- *Haematoma*—one of the most common complications experienced. Usually caused by ineffective compression or difficulty in achieving haemostasis, e.g. in patients who are obese or who have unfavourable anatomy. Most haematomas do not require intervention. Manual pressure or a compression device should be applied. Analgesia might be required. If a haematoma is suspected, the operator should be informed. A thorough assessment is required to differentiate between a haematoma and a pseudoaneurysm as the treatments are quite different.
- *Pseudoaneurysm*—occurs in the femoral artery if a collection of blood forms outside the arterial puncture site and directly communicates with the artery. Circulating blood exits the puncture site and is contained within a sac composed of thrombus. Diagnosis is confirmed by ultrasound. Management includes compression, thrombin injection or surgical closure.
- *Limb ischaemia*—suspected in patients who demonstrate a diminished or absent pulse, or a change in skin temperature, limb colour or capillary refill time (CRT). Report to the operator/nurse in charge immediately.

Vasovagal reactions

Vasovagal reactions are fairly common and can occur during cardiac catheterization, sheath removal, or hours after sheath removal. This occurs because pressure on a large artery can stimulate the vagus nerve, resulting in bradycardia and hypotension. This reaction can also occur in response to anxiety, pain, or tissue injury. Hypotension and bradycardia are often accompanied by yawning and pale, sweaty skin. Treatment includes IV atropine (600mcg) and an infusion of a plasma substitute. The volume of plasma substitute prescribed will be dictated by the patient's BP and their LV function.

Contrast medium reactions

Contrast reactions range from local allergic reactions to full-blown anaphylaxis and should be suspected in patients who display any of the following signs:
- Sneezing
- Itching of the eyes/skin
- Urticaria
- Bronchospasm.

Symptoms should be treated with antihistamines and corticosteroids. If, of course, the patient displays signs of anaphylaxis, then IM adrenaline (epinephrine) (0.5mL of a 1:1000 solution) should be administered immediately.

Renal complications

Patients at risk of developing contrast nephropathy are those with pre-existing renal dysfunction, the elderly, and patients with diabetes mellitus. Patients with deranged U&E are prescribed N-acetylcysteine (NAC), as previously discussed (📖 Coronary angiography: preprocedure care, p.139).

Percutaneous coronary intervention (PCI)

PCI is a term that collectively describes a group of procedures that aim to restore or improve the blood flow to the myocardium following a period of ischaemia or injury. PCI includes the following:

- Percutaneous transluminal coronary angioplasty (PTCA)
- Intracoronary stenting
- Coronary atherectomy and thrombectomy devices.

Since the introduction of PTCA in 1977, advances in technology, equipment, and adjunctive pharmacology have led to the expansion of interventional procedures to include higher-risk patients with more complex CAD and comorbidities.

PCI may be indicated in:

- Stable CAD
- Non-ST elevation ACS
- ST elevation ACS.

Stable CAD

Patients with stable CAD may be treated with optimal medical therapy alone, or combined with revascularization using PCI or CABG. Patients who continue to experience persistent limiting symptoms despite optimal medical therapy may benefit from PCI. CABG has been shown to improve mortality and offers the advantage of a marked reduction in the number of repeat revascularization procedures in patients with particularly complex disease, e.g. significant LMS stenosis or significant proximal LAD stenosis.[4]

Non-ST elevation ACS

Patients presenting with a non-ST elevation ACS who have been identified as having an intermediate or higher risk of adverse cardiovascular events using a validated risk stratification tool (📖 Specific principles for nursing patients with non-ST-segment elevation ACS, p.131), e.g. the GRACE risk score, have been shown to benefit from early revascularization. These patients should ∴ be offered coronary angiography with follow-on PCI if indicated, within 96h of first admission to hospital unless contraindicated (e.g. active bleeding).[4,5]

ST elevation ACS

PPCI is the use of percutaneous intervention in the setting of an ST elevation ACS (STEMI) without the use of thrombolytic therapy. Evidence suggests that PPCI is superior to thrombolytic therapy[6]; it is associated with early patency rates exceeding 90% and low rates of serious bleeding, recurrent ischaemia, and death. Current guidelines recommend that the delivery of PPCI should occur within 90min after the first medical contact or within 60min of arrival at the hospital (door-to-balloon time) (see Fig. 7.1). For patients who present to non-PCI capable hospitals:

- If it is possible to transfer to a PCI capable hospital and perform PCI within 2h, thrombolysis is not required.

- If it is not possible to transfer to a PCI capable hospital and perform PCI within 2h, thrombolysis should be commenced without delay. PCI may be indicated after failed thrombolysis (rescue PCI). Failed thrombolysis is failure to gain at least 50% resolution of the ST-segments at 90min following the completion of thrombolytic therapy. Patients who are treated successfully with thrombolysis should be transferred for angiography within 24h.[4,6]

[4] Wijns W, Kolh P, Danchin N, et al. (2010) The Task Force on Myocardial Revascularisation of the European Society of Cardiology (ESC) and the European Association for Cardio-Thoracic Surgery (EACTS). European Heart Journal **31**, 2501–55.

[5] National Institute for Health and Clinical Excellence (2010) Unstable Angina and STEMI. Clinical Guideline 94. NICE, London.

[6] Van de Werf F, Bax J, Betriu A, et al. (2008) Management of acute myocardial infarction in patients presenting with persistent ST-segment elevation. European Heart Journal **29**(23), 2909–45.

Interventional procedures: percutaneous transluminal coronary angioplasty

PTCA involves nonsurgical widening of the coronary artery from within, using a balloon catheter. It is an attempt to ↑ the blood supply to the myocardium. A balloon catheter is inserted into an artery and gently guided through the arterial system under X-ray guidance, until it is threaded up into the coronary artery. Contrast medium is injected to determine the size and location of the atheromatous plaque(s). The balloon is then advanced and inflated, to compress the plaque against the blood vessel wall. A resultant ↑ in the internal diameter of the vessel should occur, thereby improving the blood flow to the ischaemic myocardium.

Intracoronary stenting

Stents are thin mesh-wire structures ('scaffolding') that act as permanent prosthetic linings, maintaining vessel patency and keeping the artery open. The majority of PCI incorporate intracoronary stenting. Guidelines from NICE⁻ suggest that stents should be used routinely if PCI is clinically appropriate. One of the major problems with stent insertion is restenosis of the artery. A consequence of restenosis is that the incidence or reintervention is a greater risk, particularly in patients with the following[7,8] (<3cm):

• Saphenous vein grafts
• Long lesions (>15mm)
• Total occlusions
• Diabetics

Drug-eluting stents (DES)

DES, that is, bare metal stents coated with drugs to reduce inflammation or cell proliferation, have been developed to counteract restenosis. The original DES approved for use in the UK were paclitaxel and sirolimus (rapamycin); however, other drugs have been introduced: zotarolimus, everolimus, tacrolimus, dexamethasone and ABT-578 which is closely related to sirolimus.

DES are more expensive than bare metal stents, however evidence suggests that DES are more cost-effective in those patients whose risk of restenosis is greater.[7]

Drug-eluting balloons

Drug-eluting balloons are recommended in patients who have developed in-stent restenosis after the insertion of a bare metal stent[2]. During the balloon inflation, the drug, usually paclitaxel, comes into contact with the vessel.

Coronary atherectomy

Coronary atherectomy ↓ the severity of the coronary stenosis by shaving the plaque and, ∴, ↓ the size of the plaque without compressing or fracturing it or stretching the arterial wall. In theory, this sounds more favourable than PTCA or stenting; however, atherectomy is associated with ↑ complication rates.

Thrombectomy devices

Thrombotic material can become dislodged during the deployment of devices such as stents, particularly in saphenous vein grafts. Thrombectomy devices provide protection of the distal circulation. This can be achieved by aspiration of the debris or a nonocclusive filter. Thrombectomy devices are recommended during PCI of saphenous vein grafts to avoid distal embolization of debris and to reduce the risk of MI.[8]

[7] National Institute for Health and Clinical Excellence (2008). *Drug Eluting Stents for the Treatment of Coronary Heart Disease.* Technical Appliance Guidance 152. NICE, London.

[8] Wijns W, Kolh P, Danchin N, *et al.* (2010) The Task Force on Myocardial Revascularisation of the European Society of Cardiology (ESC) and the European Association for Cardio-Thoracic Surgery (EACTS). *European Heart Journal* **31**, 2501–55.

PCI: preprocedure and postprocedure care

In addition to the care described for a patient pre-angiography and post-angiography (📖 Coronary angiography: preprocedure care, p.139; Coronary angiography: postprocedure care, p.142), the patient undergoing PCI requires the following:

- Administration of a loading dose of clopidogrel or alternative antiplatelet therapy (📖 Pharmacological adjuncts to PCI, p.157) before the procedure.

Postprocedure care

Following a femoral PCI with GP IIb/IIIa inhibitor

- If AngioSeal™/VasoSeal™ is *in situ*, the suture should be cut 30min after insertion.
- If a femoral sheath is *in situ*, these can be removed when the activated clotting time (ACT) is <150s.[9]
- Following haemostasis, the patient should lie at 45° for 1h. If there are no complications and no evidence of bleeding, the patient can sit upright in bed. The patient can move from their bed to a chair after a total of 4h. Mobilization should only commence after completion of the GP IIb/IIIa inhibitor infusion.
- A FBC should be performed 4h after the commencement of GP IIb/IIIa inhibitor, to ensure that there is not a ↓ in platelets.

Following a femoral PCI without GP IIb/IIIa inhibitor

- If AngioSeal™/VasoSeal™ is *in situ*, the suture should be cut 30min after insertion.
- If a femoral sheath is *in situ*, these can be removed when the ACT <150s.
- Following sheath removal and haemostasis, the patient can lie at 45° for 1h. If no complications or signs of bleeding are observed, the patient can sit upright in bed. Bed rest should continue for a total of 3h after sheath removal and before mobilization.

Following a radial/brachial approach

The nursing care required following a radial or brachial procedure is the same as that following an angiogram (📖 Coronary angiography: postprocedure care, p.142). If the patient has a GP IIb/IIIa inhibitor infusion in progress, the drug manufacturer currently advises refrain from mobilization while the infusion is in progress.

---

[9] This may vary between institutions, so please refer to local policies.

PCI: complications

In addition to the complications discussed for patients undergoing coronary angiography (□ Complications of coronary angiography, p.149), patients undergoing PCI are also at risk of developing the complications listed in Table 8.1. Should complications occur, it is essential to inform the operator and treat the symptoms immediately.

Table 8.1 Complications associated with PCI

Potential problem	Contributing factors
Recurrent chest pain	• 2° to stretching and dilatation of the vessel (trauma) • Distal embolization of debris • Side-branch occlusion
Abrupt closure	• Arterial dissection • Arterial thrombosis • Profound coronary artery spasm
NSTEMI/STEMI	• Prolonged ischaemia, resulting in myocardial necrosis and, ∴, ↑ cardiac biochemical markers
Instent restenosis	• ↓ of internal lumen because of elastic recoil • Wound-healing process, including thrombotic, inflammatory, and cell-growth proliferation
Arrhythmias and conduction disturbances	• Vigorous contrast injection • Catheter damping (especially right coronary artery) • Induced ischaemia • Reperfusion
Cerebrovascular complications	• Aggressive anticoagulation (haemorrhagic) • Plaque disruption (transient ischaemic attacks [TIAs] or cerebrovascular accident)

Pharmacological adjuncts to PCI

When damage occurs to a blood vessel, the blood coagulates in an attempt to stop bleeding. Clotting is a complex process which involves numerous enzymes and other chemicals called clotting factors. Clotting itself activates a number of clotting factors in sequence as part of a cascade of reactions. When such a reaction occurs within a blood vessel that has not been injured, development of a clot can lead to obstruction of the blood vessel, resulting in serious complications.

During PCI, plaque rupture results from pressure applied to an atherosclerotic lesion. The fibrous cap of the plaque ruptures, uncovering highly thrombogenic contents. Exposure of these thrombogenic substances initiates the clotting cascade, resulting in partial or complete obstruction of the affected artery, in many ways resembling events in the acute coronary syndromes. The aim of pharmacological adjunctive therapy is to prevent or minimize complications (📖 Anticoagulants, p.375; Antiplatelets, p.377). In the instance of clot formation, therapy is directed towards interfering with various stages of the natural clotting cascade and includes:

Aspirin

The main function of aspirin is the inhibition of thromboxane in individual platelets. This prevents platelets from adhering to each other and to the atheromatous plaques, thereby preventing formation or extension of a thrombus. Unless contraindicated, all patients undergoing PCI (elective and emergency) should receive aspirin.

Clopidogrel

Clopidogrel is a thienopyridine antiplatelet drug, which inhibits platelet aggregation by irreversibly modifying the platelet adenosine diphosphate (ADP).[10] This has virtually replaced ticlopidine, which is also a thienopyridine antiplatelet agent, as it is generally better tolerated and has fewer reported side effects. It is currently recommended that clopidogrel should be administered in addition to aspirin for all patients undergoing PCI, unless contraindicated. The duration of administration following the procedure, depends on the indication for PCI and the equipment used, however it is not recommended for >12mths following an ACS and 4wks in STEMI patients unless there are other indications for continuing dual antiplatelet therapy.

Prasugrel

Prasugrel is an alternative thienopyridine antiplatelet drug that is recommended in patients presenting with ACS and scheduled for PCI under the following circumstances: those requiring PPCI for the treatment of STEMI, those who have developed stent thrombosis during treatment with clopidogrel and aspirin, and diabetic patients.

Heparin

Heparin is a thrombin antagonist which has been used since the introduction of PCI to prevent thrombosis. It is standard practice to administer heparin during PCI, either as an IV bolus or a weight-adjusted regimen, to maintain the ACT >300–350s, as there is some evidence to suggest that the complication rate is higher with lower ACT values.

GP IIa/IIIb inhibitors

The final common pathway for platelet aggregation is the activation of the GP IIb/IIIa receptor. Following this, the GP IIb/IIIa becomes a receptor for fibrinogen, thereby ↑ thrombus formation. There are currently three GP IIb/IIIa inhibitors available (see Table 8.2). Abciximab is a monoclonal antibody that targets this receptor on the platelets and prevents activation, and is currently the only GP IIb/IIIa inhibitor licensed as an adjunct to PCI. The exception being when a patient is already receiving eptifibatide or tirofiban, then this may be continued for up to 72h following the procedure. NICE recommends the addition of a GP IIb/IIIa inhibitor for the following patients:[11]

- All diabetics undergoing elective PCI.
- Complex procedures (bifurcation lesions, vein grafts, multiple vessel PCI).

Bivalirudin

Bivalirudin is a specific and reversible direct thrombin inhibitor which is as effective as heparin plus abciximab. Bivalirudin can be considered as an alternative to the combination of a heparin plus a GP IIb/IIIa receptor for patients not on fondaparinux.[12]

Patients receiving anticoagulant therapy are at ↑ risk of associated bleeding complications, therefore nursing care should be directed towards early detection and treatment. Extra vigilance is required at the site of sheath insertion.

Table 8.2 Indications for GP IIb/IIIa inhibitors[11]

Drug	Indication	Dose and route of administration
Eptifibatide	Patients with unstable angina or NSTEMI, who are at ↑ risk of developing an MI	Bolus injection of 180mcg/kg, followed by a maintenance dose of 2.0mcg/kg/min for up to 72h
Tirofiban	Patients with unstable angina or NSTEMI, who are at ↑ risk of developing an MI	Initial dose of 0.4mcg/kg /min over 30min, followed by a maintenance dose of 0.1mcg/kg/min for at least 48h
Abciximab	Adjunct to PCI	Bolus injection of 250mcg/kg followed by a maintenance dose of 0.125mcg/kg/min over 12–39h

10. National Institute for Health and Clinical Excellence (2004). *Clopidogrel in the Treatment of Non-ST Segment Elevation Acute Coronary Syndrome.* NICE, London.

11. National Institute for Health and Clinical Excellence (2002). *Guidance on the Use of Glycoprotein IIb/IIIa Inhibitors in the Treatment of Acute Coronary Syndromes.* NICE, London

12. National Institute for Health and Clinical Excellence (2010) *Unstable Angina and STEMI.* Clinical Guideline 94. NICE, London

Related guidance

Bosch X, Marrugat J, Sanchis J (2010) Platelet glycoprotein IIb/IIIa blockers during percutaneous coronary intervention and as the initial medical treatment of non-ST segment elevation acute coronary syndromes. *Cochrane Database of Systematic Reviews* 9, CD002130.

National Institute for Health and Clinical Excellence (2008) *Drug-eluting Stents for the Treatment of Coronary Artery Disease*. Technology Appraisal 152. NICE, London.

National Institute for Health and Clinical Excellence (2009) *Prasugrel for the Treatment of Acute Coronary Syndromes with Percutaneous Coronary Intervention*. Technology Appraisal 182. NICE, London.

National Institute for Health and Clinical Excellence (2011) *Ticagrelor for the Treatment of Acute Coronary Syndromes*. Technology Appraisal 236. NICE, London.

National Institute for Health and Clinical Excellence (2011) *Bivalirudin for the Treatment of ST-Segment Elevation Myocardial Infarction*. Technology Appraisal 230. NICE, London.

Wijns W, Kolh P, Danchin N, et al. (2010) The Task Force on Myocardial Revascularisation of the European Society of Cardiology (ESC) and the European Association for Cardio-Thoracic Surgery (EACTS). *European Heart Journal* **31**, 2501–55.

Cardiac surgery

Introduction

The most common cardiac surgical procedures in the UK are coronary artery bypass grafting (CABG), with >25 000 operations performed each year and heart valve surgery with ~8000 heart-valve operations each year.[1] Other surgical procedures that nurses may come across include surgery for AF, cardiomyopathy, and congenital heart defects. The principles of care for these operations are similar, so they will be discussed at the same time; where there are differences, these will be clarified.

In the UK, CABG has been performed for >40yrs. During this time, some techniques have changed and now minimally invasive surgery and 'off-pump' surgery is more common. Changes in techniques for valve repair or replacement have meant that those previously at high risk for open heart valve replacement now have other options open to them.

While length of stay for routine surgery has ↓, 25% of patients having CABG are >75yrs[2] and are likely to have more severe cardiac disease and other comorbidities, which can lead to ↑ length of stay, with potential problems.

This chapter covers the care of patients who require cardiac surgery, from placement on the waiting list to discharge. Although this involves the whole healthcare team, the focus of the chapter will be on the role of the nurse. In many centres roles that were traditionally performed by doctors may now be done by either specialist nurses or surgical care practitioners (who may or may not be nurses).

[1] Scarborough P, Bhatnagar P, Wickramasinghe K, Smolina K, Mitchell C, Rayner M (2010) *Coronary Heart Disease Statistics 2010 Edition.* British Heart Foundation Health Promotion Research Group, Oxford.

[2] NHS Improvement Heart (2010) *A Guide to Commissioning Cardiac Surgical Services.* NHS Improvement, Leicester.

Waiting-list management

Although some patients might require emergency cardiac surgery, most cases are elective and, ∴, patients spend a period of time on a waiting list. The target is 18wks from referral to surgery with many patients being seen in this time. There are various tools available to map out the patient pathway and ∴ find areas of delay. These pathways may be overseen by a specialist nurse practitioner. Patients are usually referred by a cardiologist for cardiac surgery, usually following a coronary angiogram for patients undergoing CABG or an echocardiogram for those requiring a valve replacement. Scoring systems such as Syntax[3] can help decide what the most suitable intervention is, however CABG is usually considered if the patient has triple-vessel disease or LMS disease (📖 Coronary angiography: postprocedure care, p.142). For valve replacement or repair, referral depends on the patient's symptoms and the severity of the valve problem (📖 Surgical management, p.91) although it is now more common to operate to prevent deterioration rather than to improve symptoms. Some patients might require both CABG and valve surgery.

In some situations, patients are asymptomatic (e.g. repair of an ASD) and, ∴, able to carry out their normal daily activities while awaiting surgery, but in most cases, the patient is affected by their symptoms. During this time, patients can become ↓ conditioned while they await surgery, which then affects their postoperative recovery. It is also an extremely anxious time for both the patient and their relatives, but this was not always addressed until fairly recently. An ↑ number of centres are now providing a service for those awaiting cardiac surgery, which might be part of a cardiac-rehabilitation programme and can include physical activities. The service mainly provides the following activities in the form of home visits, information days, or telephone support:

- Reassurance for patient and families.
- Lifestyle advice.
- Information about the forthcoming procedure.
- Symptom control.

[3] Serruys PW, Morice MC, Kappetein AP, et al. (2009) Percutaneous coronary intervention versus coronary-artery bypass grafting for severe coronary artery disease. *New England Journal of Medicine* 360(10), 961–2.

Preoperative assessment

Where possible patients are invited to a pre-admission clinic ~1–2wks before their surgery and are then admitted the night before or the day of surgery. In addition to providing patients and their families with information about the surgery, the clinic provides an opportunity for physical, nursing, and psychosocial assessments and for the patient and family to meet some of the health professionals that will be involved in their care. It also helps prevent any unnecessary delays and cancellations to surgery; e.g. if the patient has poor renal function, this can be highlighted at the clinic and further investigations organized, as necessary. Pre-admission clinics are often nurse-led and might take place in an out-patient department.

Nursing assessment

If a full nursing assessment has not been completed in the pre-admission clinic, this should be performed when the patient is admitted for surgery. The areas that are usually covered in the pre-admission clinic are as follows:

- Assessment of symptoms—how the patient usually manages their symptoms and how they affect their daily life (e.g. mobility).
- Assessment of other health problems—such as COPD.
- Assessment of hearing, sight, and language—any particular needs should be addressed (e.g. the need for an interpreter).
- Assessment of psychological state.
- Assessment of information needs—the clinic is the ideal time to address the concerns of the patient and their family, so it is important to provide information on how they can ask questions between the clinic appointment and admission for surgery.
- Check that the patient has had a recent dental examination.
- Moving and handling assessment.
- Venous thromboembolism (VTE) assessment.
- Assessment of mobility including risk of falls and pressure area score (e.g. Waterlow).
- Assessment of allergies.
- Assessment of nutritional needs.
- Discharge planning—patients should be advised to have someone at home for the first week after discharge. The nurse should also find out about any transport issues.
- Assessment of family and social circumstances.
- Pain control—a patient-controlled analgesia (PCA) system is usually used and, ∴, the concept should be explained to the patient.

Give an explanation of the surgery and postoperative care, including the fact that patients might be ventilated and sedated for a period of time after the surgery. An explanation of the intensive care unit (ITU)/cardiac recovery, with a visit if possible, is usually beneficial. It is helpful if written information is supported either verbally and/or with audiovisual aids.

Medical assessment

Patients are seen preoperatively by their surgeon, who explains the procedure, asks the patient to sign a consent form, and organizes any further investigations. The consent process should include benefits and risks of the surgery and it is important that the patient and family fully understand this. The patient is also seen by an anaesthetist, who assesses their fitness for undergoing an anaesthetic. It is common for a risk-stratification scoring system to be used. The score gives an indication of risk relating to surgical mortality and morbidity and can help the team determine which patients are suitable for 'fast-tracking' and early extubation. Most scoring systems include factors such as age, sex, severity of disease and other comorbidities (e.g. renal disease). Examples of scoring systems that can be used are EuroSCORE[4] or Parsonett score.[5]

Investigations

The patient usually has the following preoperative investigations:
- ECG—to look for any rhythm or conduction abnormalities.
- CXR—to detect pulmonary disease or an enlarged heart.
- Blood tests—usually a FBC, U&E, magnesium, thyroid function, ESR, clotting and blood cross-match. Other blood tests, such as assessment of liver function or HbA1c for diabetics can be performed as required.
- Methicillin resistant *Staphylococcus aureus* (MRSA) screen.
- Echocardiogram—for patients requiring heart valve surgery.
- Baseline observations—including height, weight, and urinalysis.
- Peak expiratory flow—as applicable.
- Blood glucose—as applicable

Other investigations may be required, depending on the patient history and comorbidities:
- LFTs.
- ABG for those with acute or chronic respiratory disease.
- Carotid Doppler imaging—for patients who have a history of cerebrovascular disease, peripheral vascular disease, LMS stenosis, or who have carotid bruits.
- If the patient does not want to receive blood products then arrangements should be made for them to donate some of their own. This needs to be at least 3–4wks prior to surgery.
- Dental examination—all patients having cardiac surgery should have a dental examination, but in particular those who require valve replacement or repair because of the risk of IE (□ Introduction, p.98).

Physiotherapy assessment

The physiotherapist assesses the patient's mobility and their lung function, including factors such as smoking history, asthma, and arthritis, because each of these factors has an effect on postoperative recovery. Patients should also be taught deep breathing exercises, which they will be required to perform postoperatively.

Skin preparation

Before surgery, any hair on the patient's chest or legs (CABG only) is removed using clippers with single-use head. The patient usually has a shower the day before and the day of the operation; in some cases, the patient uses a special washing solution, such as an antibacterial body wash.

Medications

Before surgery, some medications should be stopped. The timing of this can vary from one centre to another so local protocols should be checked. General principles can include the following:

- Aspirin needs to be stopped 7 days before surgery to reduce the risk of bleeding postoperatively.
- Clopidogrel should be stopped 7 days before surgery.
- Warfarin is usually stopped 3–5 days before surgery, and in some cases, the patient is commenced on heparin.
- LMWH is usually stopped 12h prior to surgery.
- The dose of β-blockers is halved in some centres.
- ACE inhibitors are stopped in some centres.
- Oral hypoglycaemics are not usually given on the day of surgery, and a sliding scale of insulin is usually set up for patients with diabetes.

4 Nashef SAM, Roques F, Michel P, Gauducheau E, Lemeshow S, Salamon R (1999) European system for cardiac operative risk evaluation (EuroSCORE). *European Journal of Cardiothoracic Surgery* **16**, 9–13.

5 Parsonnet V, Dean D, Bernstein A (1989). A method of uniform stratification of risk for evaluationg the results of surgery in acquired heart disease. *Circulation* **79**, 3–12.

Anaesthetic

Preparing the patient for theatre can be time consuming and challenging. It involves a team of people to ensure that the patient is fully prepared and ready to undergo surgery. Usually, the patient should be nil by mouth for solid food 6h before their surgery but can have clear fluids until 2h before (check local policy). A preoperative checklist is completed. Because the patient will spend the first 24–48h after surgery away from the ward, it is important that (if present) their glasses, hearing aid, and/or dentures are sent to the ITU to help their recovery.

The patient might receive a premedication before surgery, which is often a benzodiazepine (e.g. lorazepam or diazepam). Induction agents might include propofol (particularly in fast-tracked patients because it wears off quickly) and/or fentanyl. Central, arterial, and peripheral lines, a urinary catheter, and core and peripheral temperature probes can all be inserted after the patient is anaesthetized.

Surgery

Coronary artery bypass grafting

CABG uses a vessel (either an artery or a vein) to supply the myocardium with oxygenated blood by bypassing any narrowed or blocked sections of the patient's native coronary arteries. One end of the graft is attached to the aorta (proximal anastomosis) and the other end (distal anastomosis) is attached beyond the diseased area. The number of grafts performed depends on the severity of the patient's disease. The most common vessels used in CABG are as follows:

• Saphenous vein—in the legs.
• Veins in the arm—such as the cephalic vein.
• Internal mammary artery—usually the left artery, but the right artery can also be used.
• Radial artery—usually in the nondominant arm. An Allen's test should be performed to assess ulnar flow. Contraindications include Raynaud's disease and AV fistula.

The disadvantage of using veins is that they are more susceptible to the atherosclerotic disease process than arteries, and, ∴, may not last as long. Saphenous veins may be harvested endoscopically via small incisions near the knee.[6]

Minimally invasive surgery

Some patients may be suitable for minimally invasive surgery (e.g. minimally invasive direct coronary artery bypass [MIDCAB]). This may involve a thoracotomy approach, where the left lung is deflated and the internal mammary artery (IMA) is harvested. The heart is slowed with IV β-blockers and the graft is then anastomosed. This technique is useful in low-risk patients who may only require one graft. The drawback to this approach is that most of these patients would not normally be referred for surgery, but would probably have a PCI instead.

Another new technique is totally endoscopic robotic assisted CABG.[7] This is another form of minimally invasive surgery whereby small incisions are made and the surgery is performed using robotic arms controlled by the surgeon. The surgeon uses an endoscope via the robotic arms to visualize the surgery.

Off-pump surgery can involve a sternotomy or thoracotomy approach. Snares are placed around target coronary arteries to occlude them while grafts are sutured in place. An immobilizing device may be used to minimize movement of the heart. Endoaortic balloon occlusion may be used to temporarily obstruct the aorta instead of a cross clamp. The balloon is inserted via the femoral artery and is filled with sterile saline. TOE is used to detect balloon migration.

Off-pump surgery is felt to be advantageous because it may ↓ the risk of complications associated with the cardiopulmonary bypass (CPB) machine. This approach means that patients require ↓ time in ITU and shorter postoperative stays. However, a recent Cochrane review[8] has shown that there is no significant difference in mortality, stroke, and MI between on- and off-pump surgery although long-term survival is better in those having on-pump CABG. Some evidence also suggests that there may be higher graft occlusion rates with off-pump surgery. It is important that when patients are being consented for surgery that all the risks and benefits of the approach being taken are explained to them.

Valve surgery

Patients might have valve replacement or repair (⬛ Surgical management, p.91). Much of the care required is the same as for those patients having CABG; it is, ∴, described together here, unless there are specific differences, which will be highlighted. Other approaches to valve repair or replacement such as TAVI are discussed in Chapter 4.

---

⁶ National Institute for Health and Clinical Excellence (2010) *Endoscopic Saphenous Vein Harvest for Coronary Artery Bypass Grafting*. NICE, London.

⁷ National Institute for Health and Clinical Excellence (2005) *Totally Endoscopic Robotically Assisted Coronary Artery Bypass Grafts*. NICE, London.

⁸ Møller CH, Penninga L, Wetterslev J, Steinbrüchel DA, Gluud C (2012) Off-pump versus on-pump coronary artery bypass grafting for ischaemic heart disease. *Cochrane Database of Systematic Reviews* **3**, CD007224. DOI: 10.1002/14651858.CD007224.pub2.

Intraoperative care

Cardiopulmonary bypass (CPB)

Traditional cardiac surgery requires the heart to be stopped and the lungs deflated, so that surgeons can work on a still, bloodless heart. To do this, the function of the heart and lungs is taken over by a CPB machine. The lungs are deflated and a cannula is usually placed in the RA of the heart. Blood is then diverted from the right side of the heart into the machine. Oxygenated blood re-enters the body through a cannula in the aorta; the aorta is clamped proximal to the cannula. The machine is initially primed with 1.5–2L of crystalloid, usually Ringer's solution. CPB machines usually have the following components (see Fig. 9.1):

- Venous reservoir—blood from the right side of the heart and from suction used during the operation, is filtered to remove debris.
- Membrane oxygenator—allows for gaseous exchange between O_2 and CO_2; it can also be used to control the temperature of the patient.
- Roller pump—used to move the blood around the system and back into the body.

Using the CPB machine means that the patient's blood comes into contact with a foreign body, which would normally initiate the clotting cascade. To prevent this, heparin is administered (usually 2.5–3.5mg/kg body weight) before the commencement of CPB. The activated clotting time (ACT) is measured throughout the use of CPB, maintaining a level ~4× normal (>450s). Before the termination of CPB, protamine is administered to reverse the effects of heparin.

Myocardial preservation

Cardioplegia

Cardioplegia is the infusion of a solution, either blood or crystalloid, which contains a high level of potassium (K^+), to stop the heart. The solution can be infused either into the aorta or directly into the coronary ostia. The cardioplegia solution can be warm or cold (to help keep the temperature low and, ∴, preserve the myocardium) and can be infused repeatedly during the surgery. The advantage of blood is that it also provides an energy source for the myocardium, but it is a more expensive option.

Weaning from the CPB machine

When surgery is completed, the patient's temperature is ↑ until they are normothermic again. The heart rhythm needs to be stable (internal defibrillation might be required) and the systolic BP should be >100mmHg. Graft flow may be assessed by VeriQ system to ensure patency.[9] The clamp on the RA is removed and blood is allowed to perfuse the heart. The venous cannula is then removed. When the blood has been returned from the CPB machine and is ejecting normally from the heart, the arterial cannula is removed.

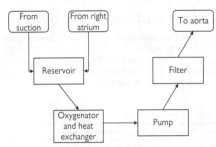

Fig. 9.1 Diagram of cardiopulmonary bypass.

9 National Institute for Health and Clinical Excellence (2011) *The VeriQ System for Assessing Flow During Coronary Artery Bypass Graft Surgery.* NICE, London.

Effects of cardiopulmonary bypass

Many of the potential postoperative complications following cardiac surgery result from the effects of the CPB machine. As the length of time that the patient is connected to the CPB machine ↑, the probability of developing complications ↑. The nurse must, ∴, be aware of the probable complications and minimize them as much as possible (see Table 9.1).

Table 9.1 Complications of CPB

Potential problem	Contributing factors
Cardiovascular	
Anaemia	
• ≤50% ↓ in PCV and serum Hb for up to 3 days postoperatively	• Haemodilution from priming the CPB machine
Haemolysis Leading to:	
• ↓ O₂ carrying capacity of the blood	• Prolonged exposure of blood to foreign surfaces
• Compromised coagulation	• Traumatic effects of arterial pump and pump suckers in the CPB machine
• Renal dysfunction	• ↑ CPB time
Hypertension	• ↑ systemic vascular resistance due to baroreceptor response (from nonpulsatile flow during CPB) and hypothermia
	• ↑ circulating catecholamines (from nonpulsatile flow)
	• Pain, agitation, shivering, and hypoxia
	• Withdrawal of preoperative antihypertensives
Bleeding	• Platelet damage
	• Heparin rebound during rewarming
	• ↓ platelet coagulability and platelet numbers
	• Consumption of clotting factors
	• Inadequate heparin reversal
	• Preoperative administration of anticoagulants/antiplatelets
	• Hypertension
Rhythm problems	• Preoperative rhythm problems
• AF, VT, and sinus bradycardia	• Electrolyte imbalance
	• Myocardial irritability
	• Atrial hypertrophy/dilation
	• Poor ventricular perfusion
	• Hypoxia
	• Hypothermia
	• Preoperative administration of β-blockers

(Continued)

Table 9.1 (Continued)

Potential problem	Contributing factors
Ventricular dysfunction Leading to: • ↓ BP • ↓ CO • Saphenous vein collapse • ↓ coronary, renal and cerebral perfusion	• Poor preoperative LV function • Perioperative MI/trauma • Hypothermia (leads to depression of myocardial contractility) • Coronary artery spasm • PEEP leads to ↓ diastolic filling • Vasodilatation during rewarming • Fluid shifts • Rhythm problems • Hypovolaemia
Respiratory *Pulmonary problems* • Atelectasis • Pleural effusion • Pulmonary oedema • Basal collapse	• ↓ alveolar distension during bypass leads to lack of surfactant production and atelectasis • Movement of fluid into pulmonary interstitium results from ↑ capillary permeability and ↑ aggregation of leukocytes • Pain and opiates cause respiratory depression • Pulmonary oedema can be caused by postoperative overload of crystalloid • ↑ pulmonary vascular resistance
Renal *Fluid retention* Leading to: • ↓ urine output • Oedema	• ADH and renin–angiotensinogen mechanism • Extravasation of fluid to interstitial compartment caused by ↑ vascular permeability, which was caused by complement activation following contact with foreign surfaces • Haemodilution ↓ intravascular colloidal oncotic pressure • ↓ renal perfusion from low CO • ↑ urine output from haemodilution
Metabolic *Metabolic acidosis*	Nonpulsatile flow during CPB generates a baroreceptor response, causing the following events: • Renin–angiotensinogen activation • Peripheral vasoconstriction • Inadequate peripheral perfusion • Lactic acidosis
Pyrexia	• Wound infection • Chest infection • UTI • Inflammatory response to CPB

(Continued)

Table 9.1 (Continued)

Potential problem	Contributing factors
Hyperglycaemia	• Altered glucose transport across cell membranes resulting from non-pulsatile flow • Impairment of cellular transport mechanism and release of insulin from islet cells of the pancreas • ↑ circulating cathecholamines
Neurological *Microembolism*	• Inadequacy of pump-suction filtration • Inadequate anticoagulation • Gaseous microembolism • Platelet activation (by foreign material) and release of vasoactive substances
Cerebral dysfunction (mild and temporary, or long-term dysfunction) • Impairment in concentration • Disorientation • Agitation • Confusion • CVA • Postoperative delirium NB: The brain is protected to a degree by hypothermia and haemodilution	• Embolism • Inadequate perfusion • Microemboli • Preoperative alcohol abuse • Length of anaesthetic and bypass operation (the risk is greatly ↑ if CPB time is >3h)
Gastrointestinal *Gastrointestinal problems* • Nausea and vomiting • Loss of appetite • Abdominal distension	• Anaesthetic agents • Pain medication • ↑ gut perfusion and motility
Wound *Wound infection* (sternal and donor-graft site)	• Bilateral IMA • Diabetes • Immunocompromised patients • Prolonged CPB time • Inexperienced surgeon • Re-operation • Prolonged ventilation • Tracheostomy • ↑ preoperative stay • Steroid therapy • Skin preparation (e.g. hair removal)

Fast-track and early extubation

Some patients may need to spend ≥24h in an intensive care unit after cardiac surgery. During this time, the patient would remain sedated and ventilated for ≤12h, while they were rewarmed and stabilized. However many patients will now be suitable for early extubation and 'fast tracking', with care delivered in the recovery area or a cardiac high-dependency unit (HDU). Some centres manage the majority of their patients in this way, managing only a few patients in a more traditional setting. In other centres, only certain patients are selected for fast-tracking. Criteria for early extubation and fast-tracking will vary (see Box 9.1).

> **Box 9.1 Criteria for fast-tracking**
> - First-time cardiac surgery
> - Age <70yrs
> - EF >30%
> - No comorbidities
> - Elective surgery
> - Cardiovascular stability.

Extubation can take place in the recovery area of theatre or a few hours after surgery. Criteria for extubation are usually as follows:
- Normothermic
- Cardiovascular stability
- Anaesthetic reversed
- Patient is alert and orientated
- Minimal bleeding in chest drains
- Respiratory rate 10–24 breaths/min
- Blood gases within normal parameters on FiO_2 (fraction of oxygen in inspired air) <0.4
- Cough-and-gag reflex present.

The patient can be given a trial on a T piece first, to ensure that they can self-ventilate without any signs of respiratory distress or change in their respiratory status.

Regardless of whether the patient is transferred to the intensive care unit or a cardiac HDU immediately after surgery, the principles of care are the same. Check all equipment, such as ventilators and monitoring devices, before the patient arrives in the unit, and set appropriate alarms or parameters. The patient will probably have the following lines and monitoring devices in place:
- Arterial, cardiac, and CVP monitoring—PA and LA lines may be inserted if the surgery is complex or the patient is high risk.
- Core and peripheral temperature monitoring.
- O_2 therapy.
- Urinary catheter to monitor urinary output.
- Peripheral IV lines.
- IV infusions.

- Chest drains (usually two mediastinal drains. If the pleural space has been opened to harvest the IMA, a pleural drain will also be inserted)—set on suction (usually 5kpa or 20cmH$_2$O).
- Epicardial pacing wires—it is usual to have two RA wires (usually to the left of the sternum) and two RV wires (to the right of the sternum, when looking at the patient).

The nurse should receive a handover that will include details of the procedure performed, any interoperative complications, whether it was on- or off-pump surgery, the length of time the patient was on the CPB machine (if applicable), support requirements such as inotrope infusions and postoperative goals, such as a haemodynamic parameters set. APPT and INR are usually checked when the patient is stable.

Many of the complications of cardiac surgery present during the first few hours after the operation, which is why it is crucial that the patient is monitored carefully. The nurse needs to carefully observe the patient for any of the effects of CPB (□ Effects of cardiopulmonary bypass, p.172).

Haemodynamic management

There is the potential for haemodynamic instability during cardiac surgery, including bleeding, hypotension, hypertension, rhythm abnormalities, and cardiac tamponade. Some of these complications can be fairly easily corrected, but some may be life threatening and require the patient to return to theatre.

Monitor the patient's BP, CVP, and HR continuously, document every 15min initially, and then hourly after the patient is more stable.

An ↑ HR will ↑ myocardial O_2 demand and could result from pain, anxiety, shivering, hypovolaemia, bleeding, a stress response, or tamponade. Observe heart rhythm for abnormalities, such as AF, conduction defects, and ventricular arrhythmias. Postoperative AF occurs in 27–40% of patients after cardiac surgery. It is more common in patients who have had valve replacements or preoperative AF. Other risk factors for AF include ↑ age, >24h on the ventilator, and COPD. Post-op β-blockers can help reduce the incidence of AF as can taking statins pre-op. Monitor K^+ levels carefully, because low levels can induce rhythm problems; K^+ is usually kept at a level of 4.5–5mmol/L after cardiac surgery. IV K^+ supplements are prescribed as required (usually no more than 20mmol in 100mL/h via a central line). If conduction problems are present, the patient might require temporary pacing via epicardial wires. An ECG should be performed soon after the patient's arrival to the unit, to check for any signs of intraoperative MI.

Parameters are usually set to keep the BP fairly low (systolic BP <120mmHg; MAP <70mmHg), to ensure that the graft sites are not put under any undue stress. The patient's BP might be high initially after surgery because of a number of factors, such as circulating catecholamines, pain, activation of the renin–angiotensinogen mechanism, or shivering. An IV infusion of GTN is usually prescribed to keep the BP within the set parameters. In some cases, other vasodilators (e.g. sodium nitroprusside) might also be required. Inotropes, such as dopamine and adrenaline, might have been set up in theatre if there was difficulty maintaining a good CO after weaning the patient off the CPB machine. As the patient warms up, vasodilatation could cause a drop in BP. In some cases, fluids or inotropes might be required to maintain an adequate BP to ensure coronary, cerebral, and renal perfusion. A variety of methods can be used to measure CO and intravascular fluid status including oesophageal Doppler monitoring, such as Cardio Q, peripherally inserted continuous cardiac ouput (PiCCO), or a pulmonary artery catheter (📖 Pulmonary artery pressure monitoring: 1, p.53).

The CVP might be slightly ↑ if the patient is ventilated or receiving CPAP. Again, parameters are usually set (e.g. CVP <12mmHg). An ↑ CVP can indicate cardiac tamponade or overload. A ↓ CVP can indicate that the patient is bleeding or is underfilled. An adequate preload is necessary to ensure good cardiac contractility.

If there are problems maintaining a good CO, an intra-aortic balloon pump (IABP) might need to be inserted. This might already have been done in theatre (📖 Intra-aortic balloon pumps (IABPs), p.350). Extra corporeal membrane oxygenation (ECMO) may also be utilized (📖 Extra corporeal membrane oxygenation, p.355).

Measure chest drains hourly for blood loss, which should not exceed >200mL in 1–2h. Do not milk or strip the tubes to encourage blood flow. If there is no bleeding in the chest drains and the patient has an ↑ HR and CVP and a ↓ in BP, cardiac tamponade should be suspected. This is an emergency and could require the patient's chest to be opened on ITU or return to theatre (📖 Cardiac tamponade, p.347). It is important to remember that while the pleural drain may be bubbling and swinging this should not be the case with the mediastinal drains.

Respiratory support

The patient might be ventilated, and if ventilation continues for some time, the patient will usually be given sedation (e.g. propofol) that they will wake up from quickly. If the patient is ventilated, this may be via the synchronized intermittent mandatory ventilation (SIMV) mode, with a respiratory rate set at 10–12 breaths/min. This mode allows the patient to take some breaths but will deliver breaths if no spontaneous ones occur. Pressure support and positive end-expiratory pressure (PEEP) (5cmH$_2$O) is usually added to help prevent atelectasis. Respiratory observations should be performed and include the following:

• Respiratory rate
• Arterial O$_2$ saturation (SaO$_2$)
• Chest movement
• Listening for breath sounds and equal air entry
• Auscultation of the chest on arrival to ITU/HDU.

Measurement of blood gases (📖 Arterial blood gases, p.62) is usually performed on the patient's arrival in the ITU and after any change to the ventilator settings or in respiratory observations. Endotracheal suctioning is performed as required. A sudden change in respiratory support requirements may indicate a pneumothorax. Immediate action should be taken if this is suspected. Those patients who develop acute respiratory failure may require ECMO (📖 Extra corporeal membrane oxygenation, p.355).

After the patient has been extubated, they normally receive humidified O$_2$ via a mask and possibly ≤4L O$_2$ via nasal cannulae. When the patient is awake, they need encouragement to breathe deeply and clear any secretions. The patient is normally seen by the physiotherapist twice daily in the first few days after surgery, but it is the nurse's role to ensure that the patient carries out regular periods of deep breathing. Good positioning to aid deep breathing is important.

Fluid management

There are a number of alterations to the fluid balance because of a combination of factors, such as fluid shifts and haemodilution during surgery. An ↑ in hydrostatic and oncotic pressures means that the capillaries are leakier, and fluid seeps into the interstitial spaces and spaces around cells (third spacing). Haemodilution occurs because of priming of the CPB machine. For the first 2–3h after surgery, the patient may have a large diuresis. However, as time goes by, this might ↓. Urine output should be ≥0.5mL/kg body weight/h. Dehydration or low CO can ↓ urine output below this level. The patient can be given an IV infusion of dopamine at a renal dose (usually 1–3mcg/kg of body weight/min), which should ensure adequate perfusion of the kidneys. If CO is ↓, address this issue to ↑ urine output. In some cases, a diuretic (e.g. furosemide) is given, either as a bolus IV infusion or as a continual IV infusion. A diuretic might be given in combination with fluids. If hypovolaemia is suspected, a fluid challenge can be given (usually ≤200mL of a colloid in an hour). Monitor the CVP carefully during fluid challenge, because a sudden ↑ indicates that the patient is becoming overloaded. While the patient is not drinking, IV maintenance fluid is given (normally a crystalloid, such as 5% glucose, as a dose of 1mL/kg body weight/h). In some cases, a blood transfusion might be required, or if there are problems with coagulation, an IV infusion of clotting factors might be required. Some centres use the Thrombelastograph® analyser (TEG®) to identify the cause of clotting problems, such as factor deficiency or thrombocytopenia. This helps to ↓ unnecessary blood transfusions.

Also carefully monitor the patient's electrolyte balance, because alterations in Na^+ and K^+ levels can adversely affect the patient. K^+ supplements might be given to prevent arrhythmias.

If renal function is normal and the patient is passing adequate amounts of urine, the urinary catheter is removed 24h after surgery. IV maintenance fluid is discontinued when the patient is drinking normally. Maintain a fluid-balance chart until the patient passes urine after removal of the catheter. Subsequently, measure the patient's weight daily, it is not uncommon for the patient to gain a few kilogrammes after surgery, which is usual, as a result of fluid shifts. This will normally right itself within a few days as the plasma oncotic pressure returns to normal, but an oral diuretic (usually K^+-sparing) can sometimes be required.

Pain management

If the patient is in pain, it affects not only their comfort, but may also alter their haemodynamic status. It might also prevent them from breathing deeply. While the patient is sedated, they will usually have an infusion of an opioid analgesic (e.g. morphine or fentanyl). When the patient wakes, continuous IV infusion is normally replaced by PCA. Perform pain assessment regularly, with either a visual analogue scale or rating score. Record the amount of analgesia used and the patient's respiratory rate, to ensure that respiratory depression does not occur. Encourage the patient to use the PCA regularly, so that they do not get peaks and troughs of pain and can comfortably move and breathe deeply. Chest drains, urinary catheter, and IV lines can all cause discomfort, so care should be taken to minimize this. Careful positioning of the patient will also help to ease discomfort. When the patient is coughing and expectorating, give them a rolled-up towel to support their sternal wound.

PCA is usually discontinued after 48h; the patient then receives oral analgesia, which will be a combination of NSAIDs (e.g. diclofenac) and other analgesics (e.g. paracetamol). If codeine-based analgesia is used, it might be necessary to administer aperients, to ensure that the patient does not become constipated.

Neurological care

Older patients and patients with a history of neurological problems, heart failure, and carotid artery bruits are at ↑ risk of developing postoperative neurological complications. While the patient is sedated, it is difficult to perform a full neurological assessment. It is common for patients to suffer some neurological problems postoperatively, such as memory loss and loss of concentration. These could become apparent some days after the surgery, but are usually temporary. It is important that patients and their families are made aware of the potential for these problems to occur, so that they do not cause undue anxiety.

In a small number of cases, patients can develop a CVA either intra-operatively or in the postoperative period. This can be ischaemic or haemorrhagic depending on the cause (e.g. emboli, heparin-induced bleed, cerebral hypoperfusion). The risk is ↑ in older patients, patients with carotid arterial disease, ↑ length of time on the CPB machine, diabetes, and patients with previous history of CVA or TIA. When the patient is awake, the nurse should perform a full neurological assessment, including movement of limbs, motor and sensory response, and pupil reaction.

A small number of patients can develop postoperative delirium which is also known as postpump psychosis. This manifests itself as confused and/or aggressive behaviour. Contributing factors can include perioperative hypoxia, anaemia, preoperative psychological problems, and ↑ alcohol intake prior to surgery. The effects of this psychosis could be transient or last for a couple of days. During this time, the patient might require sedation if they are at risk of harming themselves (e.g. pulling out lines). The situation is particularly distressing for the patient's relatives, and they need to be reassured that the condition is usually only temporary.

Psychological care

Although the patient has a number of physical needs after cardiac surgery, it is important that the nurse addresses their psychological needs and those of their relatives. The environment of the ITU and HDU can seem scary, so reassurance about the function of the equipment and alarms is vital. Although a preoperative explanation is given to patients about the care they will receive, waking up with an endotracheal tube in place can provoke anxiety, leading to ↑ BP, ↑ pulse, and respiratory distress. Steps should be taken to minimize sleep deprivation and sensory overload.

Patients and relatives can also be anxious when the patient is transferred to a less high-tech environment, because they feel that the patient is not being observed so closely. This is particularly the case when the stay in ITU has been prolonged. Emphasize the fact that this is a step towards recovery.

Anxiety and depression are common at any time in the postoperative period, but seem to occur around day 3 after surgery (the 'postoperative blues'). Initially after surgery, the patient may feel euphoric, but this can wear off, particularly because they might also be suffering from sleep deprivation. Again, reassurance should be given that this is quite normal. If the anxiety and depression appear to be severe, the patient might need to be referred for extra support and assessment. This could be at any stage in the postoperative recovery.

Wound care

The sternal wound is covered with a non-adhesive dressing, which is left undisturbed for a couple of days after surgery. When the wound stops oozing, it is usually left exposed, although this practice may vary from centre to centre. Observe the wound for any signs of infection, redness, or swelling. Infection of the sternal wound can be very serious, particularly if the bone becomes infected. In some cases, the wound might need debriding or a muscle flap might be used to replace the infected bone. As well as observing for signs of infection nurses should also observe for signs of hypertrophic or keloid scars (over healing). The sternum is wired at the end of the operation and the wires remain in place unless they cause a problem. The wound is usually closed with dissolvable sutures, but the knots on the ends of the sutures should be trimmed before discharge. Wound healing might be delayed in patients with diabetes or who have had an IMA graft.

Patients should be encouraged to 'self-hug' when coughing or sneezing to support the sternum. It is recommended that those patients with a BMI >35 should wear a sternal vest.

Bandages on leg wounds are normally removed 24h after surgery; in some cases, small drains are inserted. Leg wounds can cause problems with mobility.

Nutrition

Parenteral nutrition is normally only used in patients who are ventilated for prolonged periods. Most patients, however, can suffer from a loss of appetite, so should be encouraged to eat little and often. Calorific requirements are ↑ during the healing process, so patients might require supplements, such as high-calorie or high-protein drinks. Referral to a dietician might be required if the patient is not managing to eat within a few days of their surgery.

Nausea is common after surgery, particularly while the patient is receiving opioid analgesia. Therefore, either regular IV or oral antiemetics could be required.

Constipation can also be a problem in the postoperative period, and it is important that the patient does not strain to open their bowels. Regular aperients are usually prescribed.

Blood glucose levels are usually ↑ immediately after surgery, partly because of the stress response, but also because of impaired insulin release caused by CPB. Monitor blood glucose levels regularly in both diabetic and non-diabetic patients, because IV infusions of insulin are sometimes required in patients who do not have diabetes.

Mobility and comfort

When the patient returns from theatre, they are positioned at a 45° angle in bed, unless they are haemodynamically unstable. This helps with drainage into the chest drains. When the patient wakes up, they are sat upright to help facilitate deep breathing and lung expansion. Regular care to the pressure areas is vital after surgery, particularly for patients that are ventilated for prolonged periods. Although most patients will get out of bed within 24h and start to walk around within 48h, it is still important for the nurse to prevent any complications of bed rest. Most patients are given subcutaneous LMWH for a few days, until they are fully mobile, to help prevent deep vein thrombosis (DVT).

Initially, the patient might require assistance with their hygiene needs, but usually by ~3–4 days after surgery they are able to go to the bathroom for a wash or shower.

The patient is normally transferred from ITU/recovery to HDU or step-down unit after 24–48h. If the patient is stable, the lines, drains, and urinary catheter are removed. The patient is normally sat out of bed after 24h and begins to gently mobilize with help from the physiotherapist. The patient is usually transferred to a ward after 24–48h.

Removal of chest drains

Chest drains are normally removed 24h after surgery. There are different criteria, but they are usually removed when drainage is <50mL/h for 4h. Two nurses are required for the procedure: one nurse pulls the drain out, and the other nurse secures the purse-string suture. Removing chest drains can be very painful, so the patient should be given analgesia before they are taken out and encouraged to use PCA regularly (if applicable). The procedure should be explained to the patient and a practice run, of holding their breath or the Valsalva manoeuvre, should be performed. The procedure is as follows:

• Suction is stopped and the drainage tube is clamped near to the insertion site.
• The purse-string suture is located.
• The suture holding the drain in place is cut.
• The patient is encouraged to take three deep breaths and asked to hold their breath on the third breath.
• The drain is pulled out and the purse-string suture is tied to close the hole.
• The patient is instructed to breathe normally.
• The insertion site is cleaned and covered with sterile gauze (this may be performed at the end).
• The procedure is repeated for the other drains.
• After the procedure, the patient is observed for any signs of respiratory distress and a CXR is performed.

After removal of the drains, patients are usually able to move around and perform deep breathing more easily.

Epicardial pacing wires

Epicardial wires might be inserted at the end of surgery, in case the patient requires temporary pacing in the postoperative period. Handling of the wires can cause microshocks for the patient, so gloves should be worn by healthcare professionals. When not in use, the wires should be covered with gauze and secured. Temporary pacing might be required if the patient develops a conduction defect or if their HR is not adequate to produce a reasonable CO, which could be the case if preoperative β-blockers are used. The need for temporary pacing might be transient, but the patient could go on to have permanent pacing. Pacing is discussed in Chapter 11 (□ Types of pacing, p.224).

Removal of epicardial wires

Epicardial wires are a potential source of infection, so are usually removed 3–4 days after surgery, when it has been established that the patient does not require them. The procedure for epicardial wire removal can be found in Chapter 11 (□ Epicardial pacing, p.225).

Preparation for discharge

Patients remain in hospital for 5–7 days after surgery (although patients following valve surgery may remain in hospital for 10 days). In some centres, patients are discharged earlier than this and then followed-up as part of a 'hospital-at-home' scheme. The patient is encouraged to gently mobilize, with both physiotherapists and nurses, and is usually able to have a shower independently 3–4 days after surgery. In most cases, the patient is required to be able to climb two flights of stairs before discharge.

Factors that delay discharge

A number of factors can delay discharge or cause the patient to be readmitted:
- AF
- Pleural effusion
- Wound infection
- Chest infection
- Redo surgery
- CVA
- Combined procedures
- Prolonged ventilatory support
- Renal problems
- IABP.

Postoperative complications

Postoperatively, AF develops in ~1/3 of patients, so it is important that AF is identified and treated if it occurs. AF can be paroxysmal or might require cardioversion, either electrically or by means of medication (e.g. amiodarone). Pleural effusions, basal collapse, and chest infections can also cause problems, so encourage regular deep breathing, expectoration, and mobilization. If the pleural effusion is large, a chest drain might be required or drainage of the effusion indicated.

Wound care

Chest-drain sutures are normally removed 5 days after surgery. If clips have been used on the leg wounds, these can be removed 7–10 days after surgery; this procedure might need to be performed by a practice nurse or district nurse. However, most of the sutures used are normally dissolvable. Educate patients about wound management:
- Keep the wound clean and dry.
- Observe the wound for swelling, redness, or oozing.
- Avoid use of heavily perfumed soaps on the wound.

The sternum takes ~3 months to heal, and during this time, patients should not do any heavy lifting or twist the sternum, because this may delay healing. During healing, the patient might experience aches and pains, so encourage them to continue regular analgesia after discharge (usually paracetamol).

Driving

After CABG driving can be resumed after 4wks. Patients do not need to inform the DVLA[10] unless they hold a passenger carrying vehicle (PCV) or large goods vehicle (LGV) licence (3mth disqualification following CABG). (Check DVLA for up-to-date guidance.)

Medication

Antianginal medications are usually discontinued after surgery. The patient is prescribed low-dose aspirin (after CABG) and clopidogrel or warfarin (after mechanical valve replacement). If the patient has had a radial artery graft, they might be prescribed calcium-channel blockers to prevent spasm of the graft. Antihypertensives and cholesterol-lowering medication continues after surgery. ACE-inhibitors may be prescribed if LVEF <40% or if the patient has a history of ↑ BP, CKD, or diabetes.

Discharge advice

Before discharge, the patient and their family are educated about resuming activity, which can take the form of discharge advice talks and written material to take away. The patient might also see a cardiac-rehabilitation nurse. The advice should cover the following topics (discussed on the previous page):
• Wound care.
• Resuming normal daily activities (Table 9.2)—including work and sex (can resume sexual relations ~2wks after surgery depending on patient comfort. The patient is often advised to assume a passive role).
• Medication.
• Symptom management.
• Follow-up support and advice.

Table 9.2 Resuming activity after surgery

First few weeks	• Daily walks • Light tasks (e.g. washing up and cooking light meals) • Sexual activity
4–6wks	• Ironing, shopping, and light gardening • 30min daily walk, aiming for ≤2 miles/day • Driving
6–8wks	• Vacuuming and cleaning windows • Work (this will depend on the tasks involved)
8wks	• Hobbies • Holiday abroad

---

[10] ⌂ http://www.dvla.gov.uk

Follow-up care

Although patients may start to feel better within a short space of time, it usually takes ≥3mths before the patient feels the benefits of the surgery. Where possible, encourage patients to attend a cardiac-rehabilitation programme ~4–8wks after their surgery (□ Cardiac rehabilitation, p.325).

Some hospitals offer nursing support by means of telephone helplines or follow-up. This can be particularly helpful because there is often a lot of information for the patient to take in before discharge, and these telephone services provide a source of support and advice for both the patient and their relatives.

If the patient is prescribed warfarin, they need regular blood checks to assess their INR and establish the appropriate dose. Encourage all patients to see their GP within 2wks of discharge to ensure that they are prescribed further medication. The patient is also seen as an out-patient at the hospital 6wks to 3mths after surgery.

Related guidance

National Institute for Health and Clinical Excellence (2008) *Endoaortic Balloon Occlusion for Cardiac Surgery*. NICE, London.

National Institute for Health and Clinical Excellence (2008) *Surgical Site Infection. Prevention and Treatment of Surgical Site Infection*. NICE, London.

National Institute for Health and Clinical Excellence (2010) *Endoscopic Saphenous Vein Harvest for Coronary Artery Bypass Grafting*. NICE, London.

National Institute for Health and Clinical Excellence (2011) *CardioQ-ODM Oesophageal Doppler Monitor*. NICE, London.

National Institute for Health and Clinical Excellence (2011) *Off-pump Coronary Artery Bypass Grafting*. NICE, London.

NHS Improvement Heart (2009) *Improving the Patient Experience: Developing Solutions to Delivering Sustainable Pathways in Cardiac Surgery*. NHS Improvement, Leicester.

NHS Improvement Heart (2010) *A Guide to Commissioning Cardiac Surgical Services*. NHS Improvement, Leicester.

The Task Force on Myocardial Revascularisation of the European Society of Cardiology (ESC) and the European Association for Cardio-Thoracic Surgery (EACTS) (2010) Guidelines on myocardial revascularisation. *European Heart Journal* **31**, 2501–55.

Chronic heart failure

Introduction

Heart failure is a clinical syndrome distinguished by dyspnoea, effort intolerance, fluid retention, and poor survival. Although the management of ACS has improved, with a resultant ↓ in mortality, the numbers of people who subsequently go on to develop chronic heart failure (CHF) are ↑.

The prevalence of heart failure is around 2–3% in the overall population[1] and ~900 000 people in the UK have heart failure.[2] It is estimated that there will be an ↑ in prevalence of 50% in the next 20yrs, attributed to better outcomes for CHF.[3] The condition can occur in all age groups, however the incidence and prevalence steeply ↑ with age. The average age at first diagnosis is typically 76, with the prevalence in the 70–80 age groups, rising to between 10–20%.

CHF has a poor prognosis, the mortality rate for CHF being worse than for many cancers. It is estimated that 70% of those hospitalized for the first time with severe heart failure will die within 5yrs. However, this has been improving, with 6mth mortality rate ↓ from 26% in 1995, to 14% in 2005.[4]

This chapter will outline the aetiology, pathophysiology, and management of CHF, including considerations for palliative care. For management of pulmonary oedema and cardiogenic shock refer to 🕮 Pulmonary oedema, p.348; Cardiogenic shock, p.349).

[1] European Society of Cardiology (2010): *Guidelines for the Diagnosis and Treatment of Chronic Heart Failure.* ℘ http://www.escardio.org/guidelines

[2] National Institute for health and Clinical Excellence (2010) *Chronic Heart Failure: Management of Chronic Heart Failure in Adults in Primary and Secondary Care.* NICE Clinical Guideline 108. NICE, London. ℘ http://www.nice.org.uk/guidance/CG5

[3] Gardner RS, McDonagh TA, Walker NL (2007) *Heart Failure.* Oxford Specialist Handbooks in Cardiology. Oxford University Press, Oxford.

[4] Mehta PA, Dubrey SW, McIntyre HF, *et al.* (2009) Improving survival in the 6 months after diagnosis of heart failure in the past decade: population based data from the UK. *Heart* **95**, 1851–6.

Aetiology

CHF is a common clinical syndrome that is the end result of any structural or functional cardiac disorder that impairs the pumping ability of the heart. It is important to identify the underlying cause because this will inform the clinical management of the patient. The most common causes of heart failure in the UK are CHD and hypertension.

Other causes of CHF include:

- Valve disease (mitral/aortic)
- Alcohol (excessive consumption)
- Toxins (i.e. anthracyclines)
- Chemotherapy
- Peripartum/postpartum
- Arrhythmias (AF, complete heart block)
- Congenital heart disease (atrial/ventricular septal defects)
- Cardiomyopathy (dilated, hypertrophic, restrictive, i.e. amyloidosis)
- Hypothyroidism.

It is important to recognize that heart failure is the long-term consequence of a damaged heart rather than a simple failure of the heart as a pump. The causes of heart failure can be summarized into three main types:

- Contractile dysfunction—the heart fails to eject sufficient blood with each contraction, e.g. MI and cardiomyopathies.
- Pressure overload—the heart has to pump against ↑ resistance, e.g. hypertension and AS.
- Volume overload—the heart has to expel more blood per minute than is normal, e.g. anaemia, thyrotoxicosis, MR, or AR.

In many cases, there will be a combination of causes which all contribute to the development of CHF.

Types of heart failure

There are different types of heart failure which need to be identified.

Acute heart failure or chronic heart failure

Acute heart failure is generally used to describe the patient with rapidly developing symptoms of dyspnoea and pulmonary oedema—often following an acute MI or acute valvular problems. This can rapidly deteriorate into cardiogenic shock if emergency treatment is not instigated. Pulmonary oedema and cardiogenic shock are discussed in Chapter 18. CHF is a clinical syndrome that develops over time as a response to progressive disease, which might or might not be cardiac in origin. Acute exacerbations of CHF are a common cause of hospital admission.

Left-sided or right-sided heart failure

Patients with left-sided heart failure will exhibit signs of pulmonary venous congestion, such as breathlessness and expectoration of frothy white sputum. Patients with right-sided heart failure will exhibit signs of systemic venous congestion, such as swollen ankles and abdominal discomfort. In most patients, left-sided heart failure is usually followed by right-sided heart failure (bi-ventricular or congestive cardiac failure).

Systolic or diastolic heart failure

Most patients with heart failure have systolic dysfunction, which is evidenced by reduced left ventricular ejection fraction (LVEF <40%) and an ↑ end-diastolic chamber volume. However, some patients have the signs and symptoms of heart failure but have a preserved LVEF. These patients have an ↑ resistance to ventricular filling and thus ↑ filling pressures. These patients are said to have diastolic heart failure or heart failure with preserved ejection fraction (HFPEF). The major consequence of diastolic heart failure is backwards failure, whereby ↑ filling pressures result in pulmonary or systemic congestion. Diastolic heart failure is most common in the elderly.

Low or high cardiac output heart failure

Low CO heart failure is indicated by impaired peripheral circulation and peripheral vasoconstriction, e.g. cool and pale peripheries, cyanosis, and low pulse volume. High CO heart failure is a response to higher than normal CO caused by warm peripheries and a normal or ↑ pulse pressure.

Classification of heart failure

The severity of heart failure symptoms are usually classified using the New York Heart Association (NYHA) system (Table 10.1).

Table 10.1 NYHA classification of heart failure (ESC 2010)

NYHA Class	Severity of symptoms
Class I	No limitation of physical activity. Ordinary physical activity does not cause undue fatigue, palpitation, or dyspnoea
Class II	Slight limitation of physical activity. Comfortable at rest, but ordinary physical activity results in fatigue, palpitation, or dyspnoea
Class III	Marked limitation of physical activity. Comfortable at rest, but less than ordinary activity results in fatigue, palpitation, or dyspnoea
Class IV	Unable to carry on any physical activity without discomfort. Symptoms at rest. If any physical activity is undertaken, discomfort is ↑

Pathophysiology

CHF is a multisystem disorder that affects the function of the heart, kidneys, and skeletal muscle. Initially, a number of compensatory mechanisms develop, but these eventually become counterproductive and harmful to the patient.

The most common type of heart failure is systolic heart failure. In systolic heart failure, the heart initially responds to pressure or volume overload in much the same way as it would respond to exercise, i.e. an adrenergic response that stimulates an ↑ in HR and contractility, with peripheral vasoconstriction to maintain CO. This response cannot be sustained in the long term and will eventually embarrass the circulation because the HR will continue to ↑, but there is no reserve for ↑ contractility. Ultimately, CO will fall. Additionally, sustained myocardial workload leads to ventricular wall hypertrophy, resulting from the enlargement of cardiac muscle fibres ('myocardial remodelling'). Eventually, the LV dilates, which contributes to the continued deterioration in ventricular function.

Sustained sympathetic activity, as just outlined, and poor renal perfusion stimulate the renin–angiotensin–aldosterone system (RAAS); ↑ levels of renin initiate the angiotensin cascade, whereby angiotensin I is converted to angiotensin II. Angiotensin II stimulates release of aldosterone, which leads to salt and water retention in a bid to ↑ the circulating volume, enhance BP, and improve CO. However, in a failing heart, this only serves to ↑ the workload of the ventricle, and exacerbates the symptoms of heart failure. Activation of the RAAS also produces further vasoconstriction and the release of neurohormones, such as natriuretic peptides, which initially inhibit secretion of arginine vasopressin. Advanced heart failure, however, is worsened by ↑ levels of arginine vasopressin (antidiuretic hormone), which promotes water retention.

Considerable changes to the skeletal muscle also occur in patients with CHF. These are related to prolonged vasoconstriction and produce a marked ↓ in muscle mass (cardiac cachexia), which contributes to the symptoms of fatigue, lethargy, and effort intolerance.

In summary, initial compensatory mechanisms might delay the onset of symptomatic heart failure, but they eventually become maladaptive and contribute to the progression of heart failure.

Diagnosis

The diagnosis of heart failure is problematic because the symptoms are often nonspecific and could have a variety of other causes. This is especially pertinent in older patients who might have multiple pathologies and comorbidities. A full history and through examination of the patient needs to take place to ensure accurate diagnosis. The nurse can pick up much of this information in the nursing assessment. Close liaison with medical colleagues is crucial in the diagnosis of heart failure, especially in the 1° care setting, where symptoms might be mentioned at routine health checks. Identification of risk factors for CHD should be noted in addition to assessment of current symptoms.

Symptoms commonly reported include the following:
- Breathlessness
- Fatigue
- Peripheral oedema
- Reduced exercise tolerance
- Anorexia
- Cough.

It is, ∴, important to look for signs of heart failure; however, these are also often non-specific:
- Tachycardia
- Pulmonary congestion (LVF)
- ↑ jugular venous pressure (JVP) (RVF)
- Pulsus alternans in advanced heart failure (regular rhythm, with alternating strong and weak pulse waves)
- Third-heart sound.

Diagnosis is therefore usually made using the following investigations:
- CXR—identifies cardiomegaly and pulmonary congestion, and excludes other respiratory causes.
- 12-lead ECG—rarely normal in patients with CHF. It can indicate LVH and/or RVH, evidence of CHD and arrhythmias commonly associated with CHF, such as AF.
- Blood tests—serum natriuretic peptides (SNP can be tested as BNP or NT-proBNP) used as a "rule out" test. U&E, creatinine levels, FBC, LFT, thyroid function test (TFT), glucose levels, and lipid profile should all be checked.
- Echocardiogram—this is the 'gold standard' diagnostic tool for heart failure because echocardiography assesses the structure and function of the heart and identifies the underlying cause of the heart failure.[5,6]

Note: where heart failure is suspected in a patient who has had a previous MI echocardiography is required within 2wks (SNP is not indicated). In patients without a previous MI, SNP should be measured, if raised (BNP 100–400pg/mL [29–116pmol/L] or NTproBNP 400–2000pg/mL [47–236pmol/L]), then echocardiography is required within 6wks, however, if SNP levels are high (BNP >400pg/mL [116pmol/L] or NTproBNP >2000pg/mL [236pmol/L]) then echocardiography is required within 2wks.[5]

[5] National Institute for Health and Clinical Excellence (2010). *Chronic Heart Failure: Management of Chronic Heart Failure in Adults in Primary and Secondary Care*. Clinical Guideline 108 NICE, London.

[6] European Society of Cardiology (2010) *Guidelines for the Diagnosis and Treatment of Chronic Heart Failure: Full Text*. ℛ http://www.escardio.org

Clinical management

The main aims of clinical management are to improve symptoms, quality of life, and prognosis. This is achieved by the following means:
- Correcting underlying causes, such as myocardial ischaemia, thyroid or valvular problems, which may require surgical intervention.
- Controlling exacerbating or precipitating factors, such as overexertion or arrhythmias.
- Pharmacological therapy to minimize or reverse the consequences of the body's responses to heart failure and to treat symptoms.
- Many patients are treated by GPs, with a multidisciplinary approach to care. Specialist advice should be sought at:
  - initial diagnosis of heart failure
  - severe heart failure (NYHA IV) not responding to treatment
  - heart failure due to valve disease
  - heart failure unable to be managed at home.

Note: ♀ who are planning a pregnancy or are pregnant should have their care shared between the cardiologist and the obstetrician.

With all cases of worsening heart failure despite treatment, the cause must be investigated. Common causes are arrhythmias, deteriorating valve disease, and myocardial ischaemia. Superimposed infection and worsening renal function are also causes. Also consider concordance with the treatment regimen and any medication that might exacerbate symptoms, such as anti-inflammatory drugs.

For patients with HFPEF treatment is aimed at managing comorbid conditions, including high BP, ischaemic heart disease, and diabetes mellitus in line with NICE guidance.

Cardiac resynchronization therapy

Cardiac resynchronization therapy entails using bi-ventricular pacing to provide ventricular resynchronization. Leads are typically placed in the RA, RV apex, and the coronary sinus. This procedure can be considered in symptomatic patients (NYHA III–IV) with ventricular dyssynchrony (exhibited by a wide QRS complex >120ms). Simultaneous pacing results in a narrowing of the QRS complex and an improvement in CO. Whether this therapy improves mortality rates is still unknown, but it may improve symptoms. Current guidelines require patients to fulfil all of the following criteria:
- NYHA III or IV despite stable, optimal medical therapy
- LVEF <35%
- Sinus rhythm
- Electrical dyssynchrony—QRS duration >150ms or >120–149ms if evidence of mechanical dyssynchrony (proven on electrocardiography)

Implantable cardioverter-defibrillators

Up to 50% of heart failure deaths are associated with sudden cardiac death (SCD) and are related to arrhythmias. This incidence ↓ with ↑ severity of the condition. The indications for ICD therapy have come about from several large randomized controlled trials. NICE guidelines suggest that ICD therapy should not be used for patients with NYHA IV. It is recommended as 1° or 2° prevention.

Primary prevention

Patients with:
- Ischaemic cardiomyopathy—history of MI >4wks previous and either:
  - LVEF <35% (no worse than class III) and non-sustained VT on Holter monitoring

  Or:
  - LVEF <30% (no worse than class III) and QRS >120ms.

Secondary prevention

Patients presenting in the absence of a treatable cause with one of the following:
- Survivors of sudden cardiac arrest due to VT or VF
- Spontaneous sustained VT causing syncope or haemodynamic compromise
- Sustained VT without syncope/cardiac arrest, with LVEF >35% and NYHA I–III.

Heart transplantation

This is an accepted mode of treatment provided proper selection criteria are applied to patients with severe CHF.

Pharmacological management

Guidelines for management of CHF due to LV systolic dysfunction suggest careful titration of the following agents:[7,8]

- Diuretics—treat initially with loop diuretics (if required), and treat with K+-sparing diuretics if the initial response is insufficient (see Table 10.2).
- ACE inhibitors—first-line therapy with β-blockers. These agents improve both symptoms and survival. If ACE inhibitors are not tolerated, consider angiotensin receptor blockers (ARBs) (see Table 10.6). Consider hydralazine in combination with a nitrate if intolerant of ACE inhibitors and ARBs (see Table 10.3).
- β-blockers—first-line therapy with ACE inhibitors (see Table 10.4). These should be used for all patients including:
  - older adults
  - patients with PVD
  - erectile dysfunction
  - diabetes mellitus
  - interstitial pulmonary disease
  - COPD without reversibility.

If symptoms persist despite using optimal first-line agents, specialist advice should be sought, and consideration given to second-line treatment:

- Aldosterone receptor antagonists—consider using a licensed aldosterone receptor antagonist in moderate to severe heart failure (NYHA III–IV) or MI in past month (see Table 10.5).
- Cardiac glycosides (digoxin)—for patients with AF or severe heart failure. These agents have no effect on mortality, buy may improve symptoms.
- Hydralazine in combination with a nitrate (especially in people of African or Caribbean origin).
- Anticoagulants—in patients with heart failure and AF. For patients in sinus rhythm with a history of thromboembolism, LV aneurysm, or intracardiac thrombus.
- Aspirin—for patients with a combination of CHF and CHD, but use in caution in patient with advanced heart failure.

Recent guidance[9] also recommends the use of ivabradine to lower heart rate in those patients who have CHF with systolic dysfunction and NYHA class II–IV in sinus rhythm with a HR >75bpm. It can be used in combination with standard therapy including β-blockers.

List of drugs

Table 10.2 Diuretics

Name	Dose range
Furosemide (loop)	20mg once daily—titrated to response
Bumetanide (loop)	1mg once daily—titrated to response
Bendroflumethiazide (thiazide)	2.5mg thrice weekly–10mg once daily
Metolazone (thiazide)	2.5mg thrice weekly–20mg once daily

Table 10.3 ACE inhibitors

Name	Dose range
Ramipril	2.5–10mg once daily (may be given in twice daily doses if better suited)
Lisinopril	2.5–40mg once daily
Perindopril	2–4mg once daily
Captopril	6.25–50mg thrice daily
Enalapril	2.5–20mg twice daily

Table 10.4 Beta-blockers

Name	Dose range
Bisoprolol	1.25–10mg once daily
Carvedilol	3.125–25mg once daily (50mg twice daily if >85kg)
Nebivolol (recommended for >75yrs)	1.25–10mg once daily
Metoprolol	12.5–200mg once daily (not licensed for heart failure in the UK)

Table 10.5 Aldosterone antagonists

Name	Dose range
Spironalactone	25–50mg once daily
Eplerenone	25–50mg once daily

Table 10.6 Angiotensin receptor blockers

Name	Dose range
Candesartan	4–32mg once daily
Losartan	25–100mg once daily
Valsartan	40–16mg twice daily

7 National Institute for Health and Clinical Excellence (2010) *Chronic Heart Failure: Management of Chronic Heart Failure in Adults in Primary and Secondary Care*. Clinical Guideline 108. NICE, London.

8 European Society of Cardiology (2010) *Guidelines for the Diagnosis and Treatment of Chronic Heart Failure: Full text.* http://www.escardio.org

9 National Institute for Health and Clinical Excellence (2012) *Ivabradine for Treating Chronic Heart Failure*. NICE, London.

Nursing management: monitoring

Nursing management of patients with CHF varies according to the health context in which the nurse is working. However, the main principles of nursing management are similar despite the context:

- To monitor the patient's haemodynamic and general health status.
- To improve the patient's symptoms and quality of life.
- To enhance the patient's and their family's understanding of CHF.
- To promote self-management strategies.
- To reduce hospital admissions.

Monitoring and patient assessment

Whatever the context, the patient's condition should be closely monitored so that pharmacological therapy can be evaluated, and deterioration in the patient's condition can be noted and appropriate therapy changes can be made where necessary. The frequency of observation depends on the context and the patient's condition. Patients admitted to hospital with acute exacerbations of CHF require close monitoring because their condition could deteriorate rapidly. Assessment of the patient's general health status is also required because CHF is a complex syndrome that can have an effect on most of the body's systems. A thorough assessment can help identify any factors that precipitate an exacerbation of CHF:

- BP and pulse—to ascertain haemodynamic status. A special note should be made of the strength and rhythm of the pulse as arrhythmias are common and the pulse volume may indicate whether the patient has low or high output failure. Hypertension is a common cause of CHF, but pharmacological agents used in the treatment of CHF can induce hypotension.
- 12-lead ECG—look for arrhythmias such as AF, and conduction defects, such as LBBB, which are commonly associated with CHF. Evidence of previous MI might also be present.
- Respiratory rate at rest—patients with CHF are particularly susceptible to superimposed chest infection: any perceived ↑ in breathlessness or sputum production should be noted. Regular measurement of SaO_2 therapy is required for in-patients. Also note if the patient's breathlessness ↑ when lying flat (orthopnoea) or whether they report waking up as a result of breathlessness (paroxysmal nocturnal dyspnoea [PND]). Asking the patient how many pillows they need to sleep might help to ascertain the extent of the orthopnoea.
- An ↑ in temperature can indicate possible infection (e.g. chest infection or UTI). The temperature of the patient's peripheries might also indicate high or low output failure.
- Monitor fluid balance closely because fluid retention is a common sign of CHF. It is probably most useful to weigh the patient at the same time daily, although the additional use of a fluid balance chart may be indicated when diuretic therapy is initiated or of the patient has a urinary catheter *in situ*. When treating fluid retention, patients should have a negative fluid balance. Weight gain, ↑ dyspnoea, and swollen ankles are possible signs of fluid retention. Patients should aim to be euvolaemic and maintain a 'dry' weight.

- Nutritional assessment is required to ascertain both nutritional intake and the patient's knowledge base. Patients with CHF are often anorexic because of venous congestion in the GI tract.
- A mobility assessment is required to ascertain the patient's exercise tolerance, risk of developing pressure ulcers, and ability to get to the bathroom when receiving diuretic therapy. Patients with low exercise tolerance who are also on diuretic therapy are prone to constipation, which may require treatment. Patients admitted to hospital with CHF are usually put on bed rest to reduce myocardial workload; however, this needs to be balanced against the effects of diminished exercise. Note that antiembolism stockings are contraindicated in patient with oedematous legs.
- Assess cognitive ability because disturbed sleep and hypoxia can impair cognitive functioning, which can influence the patient's ability to engage in self-management activities. Clinical depression is commonly associated with CHF and this can also affect the patient's ability and motivation to engage in self-care.

Nursing management: patient education

The nurse should devise an educational programme for patients with CHF. Some patients with CHF will have been invited to attend a cardiac rehabilitation programme and the educational input from this needs to be reinforced. Areas to cover in the educational package should include information on the following:

- Indications of deterioration in their condition—the patient should be able to notice any symptoms or signs that their condition has worsened and know how to access appropriate help.
- Self-monitoring activities, such as daily monitoring of weight, pulse, and BP if appropriate.
- Self-management strategies, such as titration of diuretics against weight gain.
- Exercise advice—encourage patients with CHF to engage in regular aerobic exercise that does not induce symptoms. In patients with severe CHF and cardiac cachexia (muscle wastage), advise the patient to undertake upper body exercises while seated.
- Dietary advice—give patients information about a healthy, balanced diet. Advise patients to follow a low-salt diet: patients might need information on the hidden salt content of food and might also need advice regarding whether to restrict their fluid intake. Patients should be advised to avoid 'low-salt' substitutes (containing high levels of K^+). Obese patients might need encouragement to lose weight. Include advice on alcohol intake and the recommended limits for alcohol consumption, (for patients whose heart failure has been caused by excessive alcohol intake, abstinence is essential).
- Discourage smoking—referral to smoking cessation service might be required.
- Discuss sexual activity in relation to the patient's physical ability and the potential side effects of medication.
- Offer annual vaccination against influenza, and a one-off vaccination against pneumococcal disease.
- Air travel—may be undertaken if symptoms are well controlled. Long-haul flights are discouraged in patients with severe CHF. Visits to places with high altitudes, humidity, or temperatures are likely to exacerbate symptoms.
- Medication advice—in addition to education about medication for heart failure and how it works, advise patients on medication that is best avoided, such as NSAIDs.
- Driving—check with current guidelines and in combination with any comorbidities.

Palliative care

Patients in end-stage heart failure suffer intractable symptoms that require specialist intervention. At this point, the focus changes from treatment aimed at prolonging life, to the relief of symptoms. Understanding the trajectory of the disease can be difficult, and hard to predict, and differs from that of cancers, where there is a decline towards death, once response to treatment fails. Half of all patients with heart failure die suddenly, although the numbers get smaller in those with advanced heart failure where progressive pump failure becomes the cause of death.

Currently, most palliative care services are set up to cater for patients with malignancies. Although patients with CHF might not always have the same types of symptoms as those with cancer, the symptoms are, nonetheless, distressing and require palliative care. The resource implications of providing palliative care are complex and nurses sometimes find access to suitable services for their patients hampered by financial constraints.

Increasingly, specialist heart failure services are now developing palliative care expertise and can provide the necessary input. However, this is still not universally offered and is an emerging area of specialism.

Heart failure services

The NSF for CHD recommended specialist heart failure services for the long-term management of patients with CHF[10] as does NICE guidance.[11]

The management of heart failure due to left ventricular systolic dysfunction (LVSD) has a wealth of evidence behind it, however, despite this, registry data shows low uptake of these therapies in the community. Therefore there is a focus on systems of care, to improve delivery of care. There are various methods of delivering comprehensive heart failure services. They can be delivered in out-patient clinics or as out-reach, or community-based liaison services. However, the service provided is usually nurse-led (or nurse-delivered) and involves a degree of multidisciplinary input. Those who might be involved in such a service include pharmacists, cardiologists, physiotherapists, occupational therapists, dieticians, psychologists, and social service representatives.

Specialist heart failure services are designed to improve long-term management of CHF, ↑ concordance with lifestyle modification and medication regimens, and reduce the number of hospital admissions.

A heart failure service should be available to all heart failure patients wherever they are on their heart failure journey.

[10] Department of Health (2000) *The National Service Framework for Coronary Heart Disease.* DoH. London.

[11] National Institute for Health and Clinical Excellence (2010) *Chronic Heart Failure: Management of Chronic Heart Failure in Adults in Primary and Secondary Care.* Clinical Guideline 108. NICE, London.

Role of the heart failure nurse specialist

An ↑ number of heart failure nurse specialists are leading the development and management of heart failure services. Such nurses require the requisite knowledge and skills to assess the patient's condition, plan appropriate interventions, implement and evaluate complex treatment regimens, and refer to other specialist services when required. Advanced knowledge of cardiac anatomy, physiology, pathophysiology, pharmacology, and prescribing are required for such roles. Excellent communication and physical-assessment skills are also required, in addition to the ability to interpret findings from blood tests and other investigations. The future development of such roles relies on nurses being equipped with the requisite knowledge, skills, and experience to undertake them and thus continuing professional development is of paramount importance.

Related guidance

European Society of Cardiology (2010) *Guidelines for the Diagnosis and Treatment of Chronic Heart Failure: Full Text* ℘ http://www.escardio.org

McMurray J, Adamopoulos S, Anker S, et al. (2012) ESC Guidelines for the diagnosis and treatment of acute and chronic heart failure 2012. European Heart Journal **33**, 1787–847.

National Institute for Clinical Excellence (2010). *Chronic Heart Failure: Management of Chronic Heart Failure in Adults in Primary and Secondary Care.* Clinical Guideline 108. NICE, London.

National Institute for Clinical Excellence (2011) Chronic Heart Failure Quality Standards. ℘ http://www.nice.org.uk/media/D6F/93/CHFQualityStandard.pdf

National Institute for Health and Clinical Excellence (2012) *Ivabradine for Chronic Heart Failure.* NICE, London

Scottish Intercollegiate Guidelines Network (2007) *Management of Chronic Heart Failure.* SIGN, Edinburgh. ℘ http://www.sign.ac.uk

Bradycardias and blocks

Introduction

This chapter covers bradycardia, heart blocks, and cardiac pacing. Although a degree of bradycardia and heart blocks might not have any clinical significance, it is always important to assess the patient for signs of adverse effects. Adverse signs and management are discussed (□ Management of bradycardia and heart blocks, p.222), whereas cardiac monitoring and an explanation of normal sinus rhythm can be found in Chapter 2 (□ Cardiac monitoring, p.41).

Sinus bradycardia and sino-atrial node disease

Sinus bradycardia is defined as a heart rate <60bpm. Absolute bradycardia is defined as a heart rate <40bpm.[1] The causes of bradycardia are as follows:

- Vagal stimulation
- Effects of some drugs—e.g. β-blockers and digoxin
- Can occur during sleep
- Can occur in fit people
- Post-MI
- Ischaemia
- Hypoxia
- Hypothermia
- Hypothyroidism
- Sino-atrial node disease
- Following cardiac surgery
- Hyperkalaemia.

Sino-atrial disease can lead to the following:

- Sinus arrest—no P-wave activity for two to three expected beats (Fig. 11.1).
- Sino-atrial block—sinus rhythm, followed by a pause and then sinus rhythm again.
- Sick sinus syndrome—periods of bradycardia and tachycardia.
  The patient might require a combination of a pacemaker and antiarrhythmics.

If the SA node fails altogether, automaticity causes the impulse to start from the AV node (nodal or junctional rhythm). The rate is ~40–50bpm (Fig. 11.2). If this fails, the rhythm originates from the ventricles (ventricular escape rhythm). This rate is much slower at 30–40bpm.

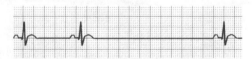

Fig. 11.1 Sinus arrest. Reproduced with permission from Myerson SG, Choudhury RP, and Mitchell ARJ (eds) (2010). *Emergencies in Cardiology* (2nd edn). Oxford University Press, Oxford.

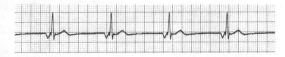

Fig. 11.2 Nodal rhythm.

[1] Resuscitation Council (2010) *Peri-Arrest Arrhythmias*. Resuscitation Council, London.

Atrioventricular blocks: overview

Conduction delays and heart blocks can occur in any part of the conduction system and might be transient or permanent. If the conduction delay occurs in the AV node or His bundle, abnormalities could occur to the P–R interval, but the QRS complex morphology is likely to be normal. However, if the block occurs lower down in the conduction pathway, the QRS complex is widened and the morphology is changed. The lower down the conduction system the block occurs, the more risk that patient has of adverse effects, in particular cardiac arrest.

If an AV block is observed on the cardiac monitor, record a 12-lead ECG to provide further clarification.

Atrioventricular blocks: first-degree heart block

The normal P–R interval is 0.12–0.20s. A P–R interval of >0.20s indicates first-degree heart block (Fig. 11.3). This is caused by a conduction delay through the AV junction. The morphology of the P-wave and QRS complex should be normal and each P-wave should be followed by a QRS complex.

Potential causes of first-degree heart block include:

- Digoxin toxicity
- AV node disease
- Electrolyte imbalance
- Following MI
- Effects of drugs such as β-blockers, and antiarrhythmics
- Hypoxia
- Hypothermia
- Hypothyroidism
- Cardiac surgery
- Ischaemia
- Vagal stimulation
- Can be a normal phenomenon.

First-degree heart block does not usually require treatment, unless the patient becomes symptomatic. Ascertain and where appropriate treat the underlying cause.

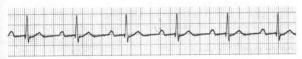

Fig. 11.3 First-degree heart block.

Atrioventricular blocks: second-degree heart block

There are two types of second-degree heart block, known as 'Möbitz type I' (commonly referred to as 'Wenckebach') and 'Möbitz type II'.

Möbitz type I (Wenckebach)

This heart block is usually confined to the AV node. The P–R interval progressively lengthens until there is a P-wave that is not followed by a QRS complex (Fig. 11.4). The cycle then usually goes back to the beginning. The QRS complex morphology is usually normal and this rhythm can occur transiently. It does not usually cause the patient to have any symptoms.

Potential causes of Wenckebach include:

- Any condition that delays AV conduction
- Post inferior MI
- Effects of drugs that suppress AV conduction (e.g. β-blockers, some calcium-channel blockers)
- Electrolyte disturbances
- Fibrotic degeneration
- Can be a normal nocturnal occurrence due to ↑ vagal tone during sleep.

Monitor the patient closely for any adverse signs. Wenckebach can be intermittent and of short duration. It does not normally require any treatment. It may be necessary to stop any drugs that delay or block AV conduction.

Möbitz type II

This heart block occurs below the AV node in the bundle of His or in the bundle branches. The P–R interval is usually normal but there are P-waves that are not followed by a QRS complex (Fig. 11.5). This can happen occasionally or there may be a pattern, e.g. three P-waves to each QRS complex (3:1 block), which can lead to ventricular standstill, asystole, or complete heart block. The block may be intermittent or permanent and this should be clarified.

Potential causes of Möbitz type II include:

- Advanced cardiac disease
- Post anteroseptal MI
- Fibrotic degeneration
- Post inferior MI.
- Transcatheter aortic valve implantation (TAVI)

It is not as common as Möbitz type I but the potential effects on the patients are a lot more serious. Refer to a senior member of the medical team if it is new onset. Pacing is likely to be required.

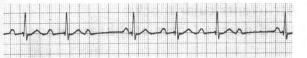

Fig. 11.4 Möbitz type I second-degree heart block.

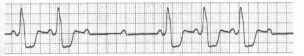

Fig. 11.5 Möbitz type II second-degree heart block.

Atrioventricular blocks: third-degree (complete) heart block

In this rhythm, there is no relationship between the P-wave and QRS complex (Fig. 11.6). The sino-atrial node is firing but the impulse is not getting through to the ventricles. The QRS rate is slower than the P rate. This slow, regular ventricular rate originates below the site of the AV block—a 'junctional rhythm' (normal, narrow QRS complex)—or lower down the conduction pathway—idioventricular rhythm (wide, abnormal QRS complex). ∴, the patient's heart rate is likely to be slow. (NB In AV dissociation the QRS rate is faster than the P rate, it is therefore not the same as third-degree heart block.)

Causes of complete heart block (CHB) include the following:
• Chronic degenerative changes
• Post MI (post inferior MI it may be transient and be fairly well tolerated. Post anterior MI it may be sudden in onset and is likely to be permanent)
• Cardiac surgery
• IE
• Aortic valve calcification
• Congenital heart block.

Third-degree heart block usually causes adverse effects on the patient (e.g. chest pain, SOB, ↓ BP) and either urgent temporary or permanent pacing is indicated, particularly if it is new onset. Monitor the patient, record vital signs, and ensure IV access is present.

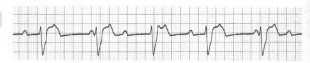

Fig. 11.6 Complete heart block.

Bundle branch block

The left bundle branch has two fascicles (anterior and posterior) and the right bundle branch has one. Either of the branches could become blocked (bundle branch block) or a fascicle of the left bundle could become blocked (fascicular block). These might not lead to any clinical symptoms, but observe the patient for any further indications of block or deterioration in their condition. New LBBB can be an indication of an MI but should be considered alongside the patient's history and symptoms ([] Specific principles for nursing patients with ST-segment elevation ACS, p.126).

Right bundle branch block

A block in the right bundle leads to a delay in depolarization of the right ventricle. Causes of RBBB include the following:

- Valve problems
- Pulmonary problems
- Arrhythmogenic right ventricular cardiomyopathy
- PE
- Degeneration
- MI
- ASD
- Any condition affecting the right side of the heart.

RBBB usually shows an RSR pattern in V1, a deep S-wave in V6, and a QRS complex >0.11s.

Left bundle branch block

A block in the left bundle leads to a delay in depolarization of the LV. LBBB usually shows an RSR pattern in V6, a deep S-wave in V1, and the loss of the septal Q-wave. Causes of LBBB include the following:

- MI
- Chronic degenerative changes
- Valve problems
- Cardiomyopathy
- CHD
- LVH
- Aortic stenosis.

Fascicular block

Left anterior fascicular (hemiblock) leads to left-axis deviation and posterior fascicular (hemiblock) leads to right-axis deviation.

Management of bradycardia and heart blocks

The suggested management of bradycardia and heart blocks is shown in Fig. 11.7.[2]

▶ The nurse must observe the patient for any adverse signs and symptoms of bradycardia and heart blocks. Not all adverse signs and symptoms need to be present to indicate heart block. Although some patients might easily tolerate a bradycardia of 50bpm, in others this could have clinical significance. If any adverse signs and/or symptoms are present, perform an ECG and a set of observations. Adverse signs and symptoms include the following:

• Hypotension—systolic BP <90mmHg
• Chest pain
• Syncope
• SOB
• Confusion
• Pallor
• Cold and clammy skin
• ↓ level of consciousness
• Risk of asystole
• Previous cardiac arrest
• Poor cardiac output—e.g. ↓ urine output and peripheral perfusion.

IV access should be present and O_2 therapy should be given if indicated. The patient may require drugs such as atropine or cardiac pacing. Pacing is discussed further in 🕮 Types of pacing, p.224.

2 Resuscitation Council (2010) *Peri-Arrest Arrhythmias*. Resuscitation Council, London.

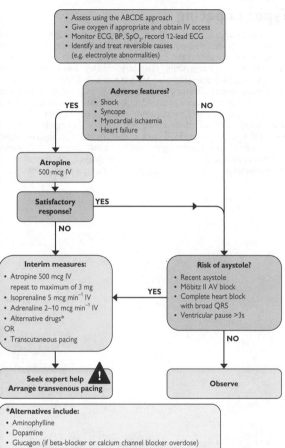

- Assess using the ABCDE approach
- Give oxygen if appropriate and obtain IV access
- Monitor ECG, BP, SpO$_2$, record 12-lead ECG
- Identify and treat reversible causes
  (e.g. electrolyte abnormalities)

Adverse features?
- Shock
- Syncope
- Myocardial ischaemia
- Heart failure

YES   NO

Atropine
500 mcg IV

Satisfactory response?   YES

NO

Interim measures:
- Atropine 500 mcg IV
  repeat to maximum of 3 mg
- Isoprenaline 5 mcg min⁻¹ IV
- Adrenaline 2–10 mcg min⁻¹ IV
- Alternative drugs*
OR
- Transcutaneous pacing

Risk of asystole?
- Recent asystole
- Möbitz II AV block
- Complete heart block
  with broad QRS
- Ventricular pause >3s

YES

NO

**Seek expert help
Arrange transvenous pacing** ⚠

Observe

*Alternatives include:
- Aminophylline
- Dopamine
- Glucagon (if beta-blocker or calcium channel blocker overdose)
- Glycopyrronium bromide can be used instead of atropine

Fig. 11.7 Adult bradycardia algorithm. Reproduced with kind permission of the Resuscitation Council (2010).

Types of pacing

A pacemaker system consists of a pulse generator (pacing box) and one or more electrodes. The pulse generator is sited externally (temporary) or internally (permanent) and is a box containing a power source, output, timing, sensing, and sometimes, telemetry circuitry. Every pacing system requires a negative pole (cathode) and positive pole (anode) to complete an electrical circuit. This provides a pacing stimulus, which is delivered through an electrode usually located in the RA, RV, or both that excites the myocardial cells, and subsequently causes a contraction. There are two types of pacing and these are termed 'unipolar' (a large ECG spike is seen) and 'bipolar' (a small ECG spike is seen). Artificial pacing is delivered in a number of ways, commonly termed 'epicardial', 'transvenous', 'external (transcutaneous)', 'percussion', 'transoesophageal', or 'transthoracic' pacing (the latter is very rarely used and only during a cardiac arrest).

Epicardial pacing

Commonly used following cardiac surgery, e.g. valve-replacement surgery or CABG.

Position

The pacing electrode(s) are sutured to the outside of the myocardium, usually following cardiac surgery, before the chest is closed. Wires are brought through the surface of the skin, usually at the top of the abdomen (subxiphoid) and attached via connecting cable leads to an external pulse generator. Alternatively a permanent internal pulse generator can be sited under the skin of the abdomen or in a prepectoral pocket (direct LV pacing for CHF).

- Distinguish between atrial and ventricular wires, either using the operation notes or by asking the surgeon directly—as a rule, atrial wires exit to the right and ventricular wires exit to the left of the patient.
- If only one epicardial wire is present, a needle placed subcutaneously in the skin must complete the pacing circuit. Use a crocodile clip connection to attach the needle to the pulse generator.

Care

- If in use, check the pacing threshold daily (☐ Threshold testing procedure, p.231).
- Monitor the patient closely for complications (☐ Complications, p.232, 236).
- Treat the site as a surgical wound.
- If not in use, coil the wires carefully (don't knot them)—protect the filaments at the end of the wire to prevent microshock and cover with a dry dressing.
- Epicardial pacing wires are frequently ineffective after their first week and most are removed during this period.
- If the patient requires permanent pacing, an endocardial pacing system is inserted before removing the epicardial wires.

Removal

- Removal is usually linked to local protocol.
- Check pacing wires have not been required for pacing for 24h.
- The patient's clotting should be within normal limits (check INR <2.5)—there is potential for cardiac tamponade ∴ monitor the patient for hypotension, pulsus parodoxus, ↑ JVP, and muffled heart sounds.
- The patient should be in bed and attached to a cardiac monitor during, and for at least 60min after, removal, because arrhythmias can occur.
- Remove epicardial wires individually using a steady, slow, downwards pulling action.
- If wires do not come away easily, they might need cutting at the level of the skin, although this can cause later problems, such as infection.
- Post removal, record vital signs (BP, HR, RR) every 15min for 1h and then every 30min for a further 1h.

Transvenous pacing

This can be a temporary or permanent system; radiological imaging will be required for insertion (with exception of flotation catheters).
- A temporary system is used in urgent situations—e.g. symptomatic CHB or for 'burst pacing' control of VT:
  - The pacing wire is commonly inserted through the subclavian or jugular vein, the femoral vein might be used where venous access is limited, e.g. in ITU.
  - The electrode(s) are positioned in the right atria or ventricle, or both (dual-chamber pacing)—connecting cable leads attach the pacing wire(s) to an external pulse generator.
- A permanent pacing system is used if the patient requires indefinite pacing—e.g. sinus node disease. The internal pulse generator sits in a prepectoral 'pocket' under the skin. Permanent pacing systems are individually programmable and the cardiologist can select the stimulus voltage and duration, sensing threshold, and pacing rate required.
  - The pacing wire(s) is inserted via the cephalic or subclavian vein.
  - Electrodes are positioned in the atrium and/or the ventricle as required, i.e. single- or dual-chamber pacing.
  - Biventricular pacing (BVP) uses three electrodes—the first in the RA, the second in the RV, and the third is inserted through the coronary sinus, into an epicardial vein, to pace the LV via its lateral wall. This is termed 'cardiac resynchronization therapy' and may improve the quality of life of some patients with heart failure.
  - Rate-responsive pacing is used in patients with AF or if a patient's intrinsic heart rate does not adequately ↑ with exercise.
  - A permanent pacing system can also be incorporated within an ICD.

External (transcutaneous) pacing

This is a form of emergency pacing often used during or immediately after cardiac arrest until a more definite form of pacing can be introduced. Many external defibrillators now have this facility. Apply the large pads (electrodes) to the chest and ↑ the voltage gradually until regular pacing occurs.

- Apply the anterior (negative) pad in a V3 position along the left sternal border.
- Place the posterior (positive) pad level with the inferior aspect of the scapula (R or L), moving it to a V6 position if capture is not successful.
- Transcutaneous pacing is often painful because of powerful skeletal muscle contractions, salt (sweat), or the position of electrodes (e.g. over bone). Patients may therefore require sedation or analgesia during this type of pacing.
- Check that a cardiac output is being produced.
- If failure to capture occurs, it is likely to be electrode position, poor contact (sweat, hair, and electrode) electricity or battery failure (note that the depletion can be rapid).
- Increasing the 'pulse width' of the device may improve capture.

Percussion pacing

This is another form of emergency pacing used for transient asystole and bradyarrhythmias or in the absence of immediate pacing facilities. Percussion pacing is most successful in very early, witnessed cardiac arrest and studies suggest some success in children.[3]

- Using the ulnar aspect of the fist, 'pace' the patient with sharp blows applied over the left lower sternal edge.
- Administer the blows at a rate of 60–90 blows/min from a height of ~15–20cm using 25% of the force applied in a precordial thump.
- This method is most likely to be effective in ventricular standstill.

3 Eich C, Bleckmann A, Paul T (2005) Percussion pacing in a three-year-old girl with complete heart block during cardiac catheterization. British Journal of Anaesthesia **95**, 465–7.

Pacing codes

The internationally recognized code for pacing currently consists of a three- to five-letter system describing pacemaker function. A sixth position for transtelephonic properties has recently been suggested. Only use one letter in each code position and always place them sequentially (I–V). The positions indicate the following:

- I—chamber paced
- II—chamber sensed
- III—response to sensing
- IV—rate modulation
- V—multisite pacing.

Since 2002,[4] the letters used in these positions are as follows:

- O = none
- A = atria
- V = ventricle
- T = triggered (position III only)
- I = inhibited (position III only)
- D = dual A&V (T&I in position III only)
- R = rate modulation.
- P = simple programmability (position IV)
- M = multiprogrammable (position IV)
- C = communication (position IV)
- P = pacing (position V)
- S = shock (position V)
- D = dual pacing & shock (position V).

VVI and VVIR pacing are the most commonly chosen.

[4] Bernstein AD, Daubert JC, Fletcher RD, et al. (2002). The revised NASPE/BPEG generic code for antibradycardia, adaptive-rate, and multisite pacing. North American Society of Pacing and Electrophysiology/British Pacing and Electrophysiology Group. *Pacing and Clinical Electrophysiology* **25**(2), 260–4.

Temporary pacing indications and procedures

The methods of temporary pacing are as follows:

- Epicardial
- Transvenous (endocardial)
- Transcutaneous (external)
- Percussion (emergency)
- Transoesophageal.

Indications for temporary endocardial pacing

These fall into two categories, either emergency or elective. The American College of Cardiology and American Heart Association (ACC/AHA) support the following acute considerations:

- Acute MI, with any of the following:
  - episodes of asystole
  - symptomatic bradycardia
  - bilateral BBB (either alternating BBB or RBBB with alternating left anterior fascicular block or left posterior fascicular block)
  - new or indeterminate-age bifasicular block and first-degree AV block
  - Möbitz type II second-degree AV block.
- Bradyarrhythmias not associated with MI:
  - asystole
  - second-degree or third-degree AV block, with compromise or syncope at rest
  - ventricular tachyarrhythmia 2° to bradycardia
  - symptomatic sinus bradycardia rate <40 bpm.

Consider the need for elective temporary pacing if patients have the potential for transient or permanent bradycardia, during general anaesthesia in the presence of AV block or for overdrive suppression of tachyarrhythmias (burst pacing only). Other sources suggest that drug toxicity, myocarditis, or hypertrophic cardiomyopathy (HCM) might benefit from temporary pacing.

Insertion of a temporary transvenous wire

- The procedure usually takes place in a designated pacing theatre because a local anaesthetic and imaging are required.
- The patient should fast for at least 2–4h before the procedure. (In an emergency this might not be possible and safe airway management is a priority.)
- A Seldinger approach is used to insert an introducer (usually into the subclavian or right external jugular vein) then a bipolar temporary pacing wire is passed into one of the following positions:
  - Into the right atrium, across the tricuspid valve and into the right ventricle, locating at its apex (VVI pacing).
  - Into the right atrial appendage (AAI pacing).
  - Dual-chamber pacing (DDD) has an electrode in both of these positions.

- Alternatively, some PA catheters have pacing electrodes incorporated in the atrial and ventricular positions and can be 'floated' into position. They are considered less reliable because wedge pressure reading can cause loss of capture.
- Check the threshold by attaching the wire to the pulse generator with connecting cable leads.
- Check on insertion, routinely on a daily basis or if the pacemaker is thought to be malfunctioning.
- The threshold may be affected by the duration of the stimulating pulse, output voltage, length of time the wire has been *in situ*, or the inflammatory response of the myocardial tissue to the pacing electrode.
- ❶ Understand the patient's underlying aetiology—↑ the paced heart rate during the procedure may be detrimental to their condition, e.g. recent MI. Similarly, patients who are profoundly bradycardic or pacemaker-dependent can become dizzy or lose consciousness very quickly when loss of capture occurs.
- ❶ Threshold testing requires a period of practice supervision to develop individual expertise and competency.

Threshold testing procedure

- Check emergency equipment is close by—O_2, suction, and advanced life support equipment including defibrillator, spare pacing box, and connectors.
- Identify the previous threshold level and underlying rhythm from the patient's notes.
- The patient should be in bed and attached to a cardiac monitor.
- Inform the patient of what you are going to do and that they may experience some dizziness—they should let you know if this occurs.
- If the patient is not pacing all the time, the sensing rate should be increased to 5–10 beats above their intrinsic rate—continuous pacing should now be seen. ❶ Ideally, test heart rates should not exceed 80bpm.
- The output dial is now turned down slowly until loss of capture is observed then raised slowly until it returns. The point where capture returns is the pacing threshold and is measured in volts (V) in the UK.
- The ideal threshold should be <1V with a pulse generation of 0.5ms.
- To ensure safety, the output is usually set between 2–3 times the threshold level.
- The threshold, underlying rhythm, and final output set should be clearly documented in the relevant patient records.
- Any significant ↑ in threshold, change, or deterioration in underlying rhythm should be reported immediately to medical staff as further intervention may be required.

Temporary pacing management

- Monitor the patient's heart function at all times, and record and assess 12-lead ECG daily.
- Patients should not leave the ward/unit, even if they feel well.
- Monitor all of the patient's vital signs, including temperature, every 4h while they have a transvenous wire *in situ* (e.g. for infection or tamponade).
- Position standard external pulse generators safely, making sure that they are easily visible and kept away from water—patients should wash but not have a shower or bath. Dual-chamber boxes are water-resistant but not waterproof.
- Protect/insulate terminal connections to prevent 'microshock' occurring.
- If defibrillation is necessary, turn off a standard external pulse generator—temporary dual-chamber boxes are shock-resistant but place the pads well away from the pacing leads.
- A spare pulse generator, with a full battery and spare connecting cables, should be available in case of device failure.
- Low-battery indicators on dual-chamber boxes require urgent attention. It is possible to change one battery at a time to maintain settings; if both batteries are removed, the pacemaker resets to its standard settings.
- The medical engineering department must check the device as soon as possible if any damage occurs (e.g. a dropped box or spillage).
- Earth all electrical equipment the patient uses and never place dual-chamber boxes near high-powered equipment.
- A trained individual should check the pacing threshold on a daily basis or if it is malfunctioning. Documentation should include the threshold, underlying rhythm (if any) and the output set. ([blank] Threshold testing procedure, p.231).

Complications

- Infection.
- Subclavian artery puncture (especially severe in thrombolysed patients).
- Haemothorax.
- Pneumothorax.
- Arrhythmias (VF/VT) caused by manipulation.
- Perforation of the RV—LV pacing is sometimes noted on 12-lead ECG because the wire protrudes through the VSD or myocardium. This can lead to tamponade. Alternatively, diaphragmatic twitching (in time with pacing) can indicate perforation.
- Failure to pace—e.g. a loose connection, a low battery, electrode displacement, wire fracture, or failure of the pulse generator.
- Failure to capture—loss or variable capture means that the wire must be repositioned or replaced. Causes include electrode displacement or damage, MI, or electrolyte imbalance. Alternatively, the threshold might need to be checked and, if possible, output ↑ ([blank] Threshold testing procedure, p.231).

- Failure to sense—the pacemaker does not inhibit when patient's spontaneous beats occur. Can be termed a 'wandering pacemaker'. Causes include wire damage, an incorrect sensing threshold, poor positioning, or equipment failure.
- Pacemaker dependence—the patient's intrinsic heart rate becomes insufficient to sustain life (e.g. asystole).

Removal of temporary wire(s)

- The patient should be in bed, in either a supine or modified-Trendelenburg position. ▶ There is a risk of air embolism with any central venous access.
- The procedure is aseptic. ▶ The external wire can be sutured into place.
- Patients should be cardiac monitored because the myocardium can be irritated by wire removal, e.g. RV wires must pass through the tricuspid valve and this can cause arrhythmias.
- A defibrillator should be available.
- If any resistance is felt, contact the medical team to remove the wire under radiographic guidance.
- After removal, cover the site with an air-occlusive dressing, which should remain *in situ* for at least 24h to enable healing at the entry site.
- Frequently, the tip of the wire is sent for M,C&S, and patient is treated accordingly.
- Patients should be cardiac monitored—telemetry might be appropriate.
- Record vital signs regularly for 48h; recording the patient's temperature every 4h is also recommended.
- Observe the site for leakage (blood) or swelling and then redness or other signs of infection.

Permanent pacing indications and procedures

Indications

- Heart blocks:
  - sino-atrial block
  - Möbitz type II
  - third-degree (CHB)
  - trifasicular block
  - congenital heart block.
- Symptomatic bradycardia (unresponsive to other treatment).
- Sick sinus syndrome (abnormal SA node function) and/or AV block.
- Ventricular standstill.
- Neurally mediated syncope (tilt test diagnosis)—dual-chamber pacing is beneficial in some patients.
- HCM (usually temporary pacing trial first, but not all patients benefit).
- Dilated cardiomyopathy, congestive heart failure—BVP/LV pacing.
- Long QT syndrome.
- Drug-refractory paroxysmal AF (multisite pacing).
- 'Tachy–brady' (sick sinus) syndrome.

Procedures

Patient preparation

- Assess the patient to focus on individual needs before insertion of a permanent pacing system. Patient education, including preprocedure and postprocedure information, is discussed elsewhere (📖 Education of paced patients, p.238).
- Implantation occurs under local anaesthetic ∴ prepare patients for a surgical procedure—e.g. ensure correct identification, informed consent, NBM, and IV hydration.
- Patients are normally prescribed systematic prophylactic antibiotics and premedication.
- The nondominant side is usually chosen for the pulse generator site, although it might not always be appropriate (e.g. after mastectomy). Keep it free from ECG electrode placement, and locate IV access opposite the insertion site for easier access during the procedure.
- The procedure is performed aseptically in a pacing theatre or cardiac catheter laboratory, although bedside insertion can occur if mobile fluoroscopy is available.
- Patients are awake during the procedure so inform them of any staff present to minimize stress; keep noise or disturbance to a minimum.
- Electrodes are introduced through the cephalic or subclavian vein and usually sited in the right atrial appendage or right ventricular apex, or both (multisite pacing is also used).
- The internal pulse generator is inserted into a prepectoral 'pocket'.
- A technician usually performs a pacemaker 'check', which should be documented in the patient's notes.

Post procedure

- Closely monitor the patient in a CCU/HDU.
- Be aware of the type of device inserted, the pacing mode, rate limits set, and whether a CXR (usually PA and lateral) has been performed and assessed post insertion.
- The patient should be continuously cardiac monitored (use the 'pacing on' function) to establish rhythm and detect pacing irregularities. Also, record a 12-lead ECG.
- Regularly record vital signs—every 30min for 2h, every 1h for the next 2h and then as necessary. Assess temperature every 4h during the patient's hospital stay to detect infection.
- Patients who are breathless and experience pain on inspiration could have a pneumothorax or haemothorax (□ Complications, p.236), which requires urgent medical intervention (chest drain).
- The early wound assessment is for bleeding or haematoma formation—the latter can sometimes develop over a period of several hours before detection.
- Ongoing wound assessment should identify redness, swelling, oozing, or other signs of infection.
- Prescribe patients oral analgesia for discomfort—the local anaesthetic administered during the procedure seems to limit significant postprocedure pain in many patients.
- Advise patients to minimize arm movements on the affected side, to prevent wire displacement (this is less likely if a 'screw-in' electrode is used).

Permanent pacing management

Patients who have a permanent pacemaker that is working effectively should require minimal management.

- Specific patient education (Education of paced patients, p.238).
- Patients must carry a pacemaker registration card and alert doctors or dentists to this before any procedure.
- Follow-up appointments are scheduled every 3–12mths, depending on the type of pacemaker and problems experienced. The patient's health and pacemaker function are checked at these appointments.
- The battery life varies (between 6–10yrs) and patients need more frequent pacing checks and a 'box change' towards the end of the battery's life.

There are a number of clinical situations that might need specific management:

- Defibrillation (emergency or elective)—keep paddles/pads well away from the pulse generator and check the pacemaker function following the procedure (as appropriate).
- Diathermy can cause inappropriate inhibition, VF, or VT. Paced patients must be cardiac monitored throughout any surgical procedure.
- Patients must never receive or be in close proximity to MRI scanning.
- Radiotherapy can damage pacemaker circuitry so shield the area during treatment. If the pulse generator is in direct conflict with the area being treated, it will need to be moved.
- Magnet use for assessment of function. Magnets near or over the pulse generator convert pacing to a 'fixed mode', which can be useful in diagnosing sensing problems, aiding testing if the patient is in their own rhythm or where electromagnetic interference can inhibit output.

Complications

- Pneumothorax/haemothorax—can occur during implantation or in the immediate postoperative period. Affected patients usually require a chest drain. Check ↑ respiratory rate, depth, ease, pain, auscultatory and percussion changes, tracheal deviation, and CXR.
- Bleeding/haematoma—expect some bruising. Patients who have AF or artificial heart valves requiring concomitant anticoagulation need careful monitoring before, during, and following the procedure.
- Pericardial effusion/tamponade—a perforated pacing wire could be the cause, occurring during or after the procedure.
- Wire displacement—usually occurs in the first few hours and the patient requires a second procedure to reattach the detached wire. Failure to pace, sense, or capture might be seen on the ECG. Minimizing arm movements might limit occurrence.
- Infection—can occur at any time post insertion. Advise patients of its signs and symptoms and the need to contact their pacemaker clinic urgently (Long-term management of paced patients, p.240).
- Vein thrombosis—occurs during the first few days and patients might present with a swollen arm or neck, or discolouration of their hand or arm. Veins around the affected area might be engorged. Treatment is dependent on the vein affected.

- Erosion—usually occurs after several months, often in thinner patients. It requires pulse generator relocation and there might be an associated infection to treat.
- Pacemaker dependency—the patient is totally dependent on their pacemaker and has little or no intrinsic heart rate (e.g. asystole).
- Pacemaker syndrome—patients experience congestive signs and symptoms due to retrograde conduction and may have more than a 20mmHg drop in BP when paced. This leads to syncope, dizziness, dyspnoea, and malaise. It is usually experienced in single-chamber ventricular pacing. NICE have provided specific guidance on the use of dual-chamber pacing for sick sinus and atrioventricular block.[5]
- Failure to pace, sense, capture (☐ Temporary pacing management, p.232).
- Patient manipulation of the pulse generator can cause lead displacement/damage.
- Cardiac arrest, allergic reaction, or death.

[5] National Institute for Health and Clinical Excellence (2005) *Dual-chamber Pacemakers for Symptomatic Bradycardia Due to Sick Sinus Syndrome and/or Atrioventricular Block.* NICE, London.

Education of paced patients

Preoperative

Patients should be aware that the pacemaker does not cure heart disease, although it might significantly improve their lifestyle. Discussion should include explanation of the following:

- The patient's specific problem.
- The type of device, why it is needed, what it will do, and how and where it will be inserted.
- Immediate postoperative care, discharge planning, and the need for long-term follow-up (📖 Long-term management of paced patients, p.240).
- If they are an out-patient, inform the patient of the local policy for taking their medication before admission. For example, clopidogrel (stop 5 days before admission), warfarin (INR should be >2 for 4wks then checked 3 days before admission). Note that some patients might be admitted early for IV heparin control.

Postoperative

- Patients receive a letter for their GP and district nurse detailing the procedure and aftercare, with advice regarding suture removal (if used).
- Shoulder exercises—patients must have physiotherapy advice to prevent 'frozen shoulder' occurring as a result of their restricted range of arm movement during the first week.
- If there is any return of fainting, dizziness, palpitations, or development of pain, tenderness, swelling, fever, or wound discharge, the patient must contact their pacing clinic urgently—if symptoms occur 'out of hours', they should contact their GP service or Minor Injuries Unit or, and if symptoms are acute, they should contact the emergency services.
- MedicAlert—UK patients can be given advice on how to join 'Medic Alert', which enables health professionals anywhere in the world to check patient information.
- Driving—2011 guidance states that all UK patients must inform the DVLA and can drive a car or motorcycle 1wk after pacemaker insertion or box change with a normal licence (exceptions include post MI, cardiac surgery, and epilepsy). Holders of an LGV or PSV licence cannot drive these vehicles for 6wks after pacemaker insertion. All patients must attend regular pacing checks and have no other exclusions from driving.
- Sport—normally resumed after 3–4wks, although greater care is advised for 'contact' sports.
- Proximity of magnetic devices:
  - Well-maintained household tools/machines do not present a risk.
  - Mobile phones—keep at least 15cm away from the pacemaker. Do not store the phone in the breast pocket and try to use the opposite ear.

- Ultrasonic dental cleaners—dentists and hygienists can use traditional instruments to clean and polish teeth.
- Airports, libraries, and shops with security devices—if it is necessary to pass through these, do so quickly and then move well away. Always carry a patient registration card.
- Return to work—advice is nonspecific. However, jobs that require heavy lifting (e.g. the building trade) or use strong magnetic devices (e.g. arc welding) require a longer period of recuperation and sometimes cannot be resumed.
- All patients should attend regular follow-up appointments for life.

Long-term management of paced patients

Pacing clinics

Clinical guidance provides the following aims for pacing clinics:

- To ensure the best possible function of the pacing system, incorporating the patient's needs with safe maximization of the pulse generator's life.
- To identify any abnormalities or complications of pacing and provide prompt therapeutic intervention.
- The prediction of the end of the pulse generator's life, enabling elective (non-urgent) change of the pulse generator.
- To provide patient support and education and training opportunities for medical and paramedical staff.
- To maintain a database of information on current and previous pacing systems for each patient.
- To collate general data on the function of pulse generators.
- To provide a clinical cardiology follow-up service, as appropriate.

The Healthcare Quality Improvement Partnership continues the drive to audit practice. Their Heart Rhythm Management Project monitors activities and trends in pacing.

Box replacement

- Patients are admitted every 6–10yrs for replacement of the pulse generator that houses the battery.
- Regular visits to the pacing clinic will identify the end of the pulse generator's life and arrange elective replacement.
- The procedure requires a local anaesthetic, as for insertion.
- Existing transvenous pacing wires are usually left *in situ* if they are functioning correctly.
- The new pulse generator is attached and placed into the existing pocket under the skin.
- If the patient is pacemaker-dependent, a temporary pacing system is inserted, usually through the femoral vein for use while the permanent system is changed.
- A box change might also be indicated in 'pacemaker syndrome'.

Related guidance

Cunningham D, Charles R, Cunningham M, de Lange A (2011) *Cardiac Rhythm Management: UK National Clinical Audit 2010*. The National Institute for Cardiovascular Outcomes Research, London.

Dretzke J, Toff W, Lip G, Raftery J, Fry-Smith A, Taylor R (2004, published online 2009) Dual chamber versus single chamber ventricular pacemakers for sick sinus syndrome and atrioventricular block. *Cochrane Database of Systematic Reviews* **2**, CD003710. DOI: 10.1002/14651858. CD003710.pub2.

Heart Rhythm UK (2011) *Standards for Implantation and Follow-up of Cardiac Rhythm Management Devices*. Heart Rhythm UK, London.

Resuscitation Council UK (2010) *Peri-Arrest Arrhythmias*. Resuscitation Council, London.

Vardas PE, Auricchio A, Blanc JJ, et al. (2007) Guidelines for cardiac pacing and cardiac resynchronization therapy. *European Heart Journal* **28**, 2256–95.

Tachycardias

Introduction

This chapter looks at the diagnosis and management of tachycardias, including both narrow complex tachycardias and broad complex tachycardias. Atrial fibrillation (AF) is the most common sustained arrhythmia, affecting 1–2% of the general population (5–15% of those >80yrs).[1] There have been a number of developments in arrhythmia care over the last few years in particular in relation to AF and there are now more specialist arrhythmia nurses and nurse-led arrhythmia services than ever before. AF, arrhythmias, and sudden cardiac death (SCD) are priority areas of NHS improvement.

[1] The Task Force of the European Society of Cardiology (2010) Guidelines for the management of atrial fibrillation. *European Heart Journal* **31**, 2369–429.

Supraventricular tachycardia

Supraventricular tachycardia (SVT) is an umbrella term given to all tachy-cardias originating above the ventricles, e.g. atrial tachycardia, atrial flutter, and AF. However, many people associate SVT with atrial tachycardia.

Atrial tachycardia usually results from either enhanced automaticity or a re-entry circuit. The characteristics of atrial tachycardia are as follows:
• Rate usually 140–220bpm.
• P-wave morphology might be different or P-waves might be absent.
• Usually responds to carotid sinus massage (CSM).
• Can occur in healthy individuals.
• Usually starts and stops abruptly.

The causes of atrial tachycardia include alcohol, stress, nicotine, caffeine, lung disease, medical or recreational drugs, PE, and CHD.

Re-entry tachycardia

There are two main types of re-entry tachycardia:
• Atrioventricular node re-entry tachycardia (AVNRT; Fig. 12.1)—caused by re-entry circuits within the AV node.
• Atrioventricular re-entry tachycardia (AVRT)—caused by accessory pathways.

Of the two types, AVNRT is the commonest. It might be difficult to dis-tinguish between the two types on an ECG or rhythm strip; however, if the P-wave is hidden, it is considered more likely to be AVNRT, and if it is following the QRS, then it is more likely to be AVRT. Atrial flutter with a 2:1 block can also look like atrial tachycardia. If CSM is performed on a person with atrial flutter, the ventricular rate usually slows and the flutter waves become more evident.

AVNRT

There might be dual pathways within the AV node that have different rates of conductivity and refractoriness. ∴, an impulse could pass down one pathway and set up a re-entry circuit by going up the other pathway. This can lead to retrograde atrial depolarization. It usually starts and stops abruptly and can last seconds, hours, or, in less common cases, days. The patient might experience dyspnoea, palpitations, dizziness, chest pain, and polyuria. The management of AVNRT includes the following:
• Observations.
• Record an ECG. This may have already been recorded either pre hospital or in the A&E department.
• Holter monitoring.
• Investigation into the precipitating factors.
• Vagal manoeuvres (Box 12.1).
• Electrophysiology studies (EPS) (📖 Basic electrophysiology, p.263).
• Drugs such as adenosine, amiodarone, and β-blockers.
• In some cases, catheter ablation (📖 Ablation, p.269).

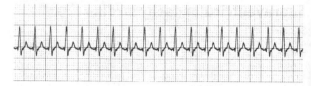

Fig. 12.1 Atrioventricular node re-entry tachycardia.

Box 12.1 Types of vagal manoeuvre

1. Valsalva manoeuvre—instruct the patient to take a deep breath and hold it. They can either blow out against closed lips or put their thumb tip in their mouth and blow against it for ~20s. The patient should be sitting or lying down.
2. CSM—massage the carotid artery for ~15s. Do not perform this on elderly patients or those with a history of CVA, TIA, carotid bruits, or arterial disease.
3. Diving reflex—immerse the patient's face in icy water for ~1–2s.
4. Induce gagging.
5. Swallow ice cold water.

NB—All of these manoeuvres should only be done under close supervision.

AVRT

The most well-known cause of AVRT is Wolff–Parkinson–White syndrome (WPW). An accessory pathway between the atria and ventricles (usually on the left side) enables the impulse from the SA node to cause early activation of part of the ventricle. The rest of the ventricles are depolarized in the normal fashion. This leads to the following characteristics:

- Shortened P–R interval (<0.12s)
- Delta (δ)-wave
- Widened QRS complex (>0.12s).

Orthodromic AVRT is the most common form, in which the impulse travels from the atria to the ventricles via the AV node and then back up via the accessory pathway. The ECG does not show the usual characteristics of WPW. If, however, the conduction is antidromic, the impulse travels from the atria to the ventricles via the accessory pathway and then back up via the AV node. The ECG shows δ-waves and broad QRS complexes. Although WPW might not cause a problem for many people, atrial fibrillation in the presence of WPW can be dangerous because the impulses can travel down the accessory pathway and cause VF.

The management of WPW is similar to that described for AVNRT. However, treatment with verapamil or digoxin should be avoided particularly in those who have a history of WPW with AF as these can block AV node conduction.

Atrial fibrillation

AF (Fig. 12.2) is the most common sustained arrhythmia and results from either multiple re-entry circuits or irregular depolarization within the atria. AF can lead to a doubling of mortality rate, ↑ risk of heart failure, stroke, and poor quality of life. Therefore identification of those in AF through a simple pulse check is very important. The characteristics of AF are as follows:

- Chaotic baseline
- Atrial rate >300bpm/min
- No clearly identifiable P-wave
- Normal QRS complex width and morphology (usually)
- Irregular QRS rate
- Irregular pulse
- Risk of thrombus.

AF has been classified[2] as:

- First episode—presenting for the first time.
- Paroxysmal—terminates spontaneously within 48h but paroxysms may continue for up to 7 days.
- Persistent—episode lasting >7 days but responds to pharmaceutical or electrical cardioversion.
- Long-standing persistent—AF of 1 year or more, rhythm control strategy adopted.
- Permanent—AF accepted by patient and clinician.

There are many causes of AF, and although it does usually occur in the presence of heart disease, in younger patients there might be no apparent cause (lone AF). Causes of AF include the following:

- Alcohol
- MI
- Cardiac surgery
- Electrolyte imbalance
- Anaemia
- Hypoxaemia
- ↑ BP
- Congenital
- ↑ age
- Thyrotoxicosis
- Valve disorders (particularly mitral valve disorders)
- LAH
- Heart failure
- Cardiomyopathy
- Lone AF—no history of cardiovascular disease or hypertension. No abnormal cardiac signs, normal CXR, and ECG (apart from AF).

The effects of AF can vary from quite mild in permanent AF with a controlled ventricular response to quite severe. Classification of AF-related symptoms can be done using the EHRA score.[2] Effects of AF include the following:

- SOB
- Chest pain
- Hypotension
- Palpitations
- ↓ CO

- Emboli
- Loss of AV filling.

There are many different treatment options for AF,[2] which depend on the stroke risk, ventricular rate, and the effects of AF on the patient. The goals of treatment are to ↓ risk of stroke, rate and/or rhythm control, and avoid adverse effects.

If the patient is experiencing AF with a rapid ventricular response, the nurse should perform a set of cardiovascular observations and record an ECG. The patient might require O₂ therapy. An Echo may be performed to assess for underlying structural heart problems.

General management of arrhythmias is discussed (📖 Management of tachycardias, p.254), but the management of AF could include the following:
- Managing and treating the cause.
- Electrical (direct current [DC]) cardioversion. DC cardioversion is particularly used in patients who are haemodynamically unstable (📖 Direct current cardioversion, p.256). Anticoagulation should be given for 3wks prior to cardioversion in AF >24h.
- Pharmacological cardioversion—e.g. amiodarone, dronedarone, flecainide, and some β-blockers.
- Rate control—e.g. digoxin, β-blockers.
- In some cases pacing or catheter or surgical ablation (📖 Ablation, p.269) may be used as treatment options.

Stroke prevention

There are a number of tools that can be used to assess the risk of stroke and the risks/benefits of anticoagulation including: GRASP AF,[3] CHA₂DS₂-VASc,[4] and HAS-BLED.[5] Anticoagulation should be given unless risks outweigh the benefits. This would normally be warfarin but newer drugs such as dabigatran or rivaroxaban may be used. Left atrial appendage excision or left atrial occlusion can be performed on those patients who have a high risk of thromboembolic stroke but in whom warfarin is contraindicated.

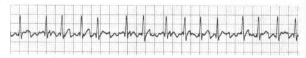

Fig. 12.2 Atrial fibrillation.

[2] The Task Force of the European Society of Cardiology (2010) Guidelines for the management of atrial fibrillation. *European Heart Journal* **31**, 2369–429.

[3] NHS Improvement (2009) *Guidance on Risk Assessment and Stroke Prevention for Atrial Fibrillation (GRASP-AF).* ℘ http://www.improvement.nhs.uk/graspaf (accessed 11 February 2012).

[4] Lip GY, Frison L, Halperin JL, Lane DA (2010) Identifying patients at high risk for stroke despite anticoagulation. *Stroke* **41**, 2731–8.

[5] Pisters R, Lane DR, Nieuwlaat R, de vos CB, Crijins HJ, Lip GYH (2010) A novel user friendly score (HAS-BLED) to assess one year risk of major bleeding in atrial fibrillation patients – European Heart Survey. *Chest.* **138**, 1093–100.

Atrial flutter

Atrial flutter (Fig. 12.3) is less common than AF. It usually arises from a re-entry circuit within the RA. The characteristics of atrial flutter are as follows:
- Atrial rate of 250–400bpm/min.
- Flutter waves are present.
- There is usually an AV block of 2:1, 3:1, 4:1, and so forth.
- Regularity and AV block can vary.
- CSM usually ↑ block and rarely converts the person to sinus rhythm.

The causes of atrial flutter are similar to AF and include the following:
- Rheumatic heart disease
- CHD
- LAH
- ASD.

β-blockers can be given to try and prevent atrial flutter occurring, but in general medications are less successful at treating atrial flutter than cardioversion. Ablation may also be used. Anticoagulation should be given to those at risk of thromboembolic events.

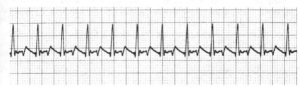

Fig. 12.3 Atrial flutter.

Ventricular rhythms

Ventricular rhythms can result from escape, enhanced automaticity, ectopic foci, and re-entry circuits. They are usually considered to be more life threatening than supraventricular rhythms because they can cause cardiac arrest and death.

Ventricular ectopics (VE) can occur in a normal heart but could also be a sign of a poor LV function. They can occur following MI and could be caused by electrolyte disturbances, ischaemia, or necrosis and ↓ oxygen levels. They do not usually require treatment, although it is usually wise to check the K$^+$ levels of the patient if these are not known. Some of the characteristics of VE are as follows:

- Bizarre looking and wide QRS complex (width >0.12s).
- No obvious P-wave.
- Compensatory pause.
- They can be unifocal, multifocal (different morphology) and occur every other sinus beat (bigeminy) or together in twos and threes (couplets and salvos).

If an ectopic falls on the vulnerable part of a T-wave, this can precipitate VF (R-on-T phenomenon).

Accelerated idioventricular rhythm

Although this is not considered to be a serious arrhythmia, it can occur as a result of enhanced automaticity or a failure of the conduction system higher up the pathway. It is most commonly seen following thrombolysis for STEMI. It is not usually treated if the patient is haemodynamically stable. Its characteristics are as follows:

- A ventricular rate of 50–110bpm
- Wide QRS complex (no P-wave)
- Similar to ventricular escape rhythm.

Ventricular tachycardia

Pulseless ventricular tachycardia (Fig. 12.4) is one of the cardiac arrest rhythms and should be treated with immediate DC shock and managed using the ALS algorithm (☐ Advanced life support, p.341). In some cases, however, people might have short episodes of VT with a pulse. These can be self-terminating. VT is characterized by QRS complexes that are >0.12s in width. An independent P-wave might be seen. VT can be monomorphic (one focus) or polymorphic.

If a patient goes into VT, it is vital that they are monitored and that their haemodynamic status is checked. The patient can easily lose their cardiac output and could ultimately lose consciousness and suffer a cardiac arrest. The acute management of VT (with a pulse) is discussed in Chapter 12 (☐ Management of tachycardias, p.254). For those people who develop recurrent episodes of VT, an internal cardiac defibrillator might need to be inserted (☐ Implantable cardioverter-defibrillators, p.257) or in some cases ablation may be suitable (☐ Ablation, p.269). The NICE guidelines[6] suggest that patients who suffer haemodynamic compromise (↓ BP, LVF, and chest pain) or those without haemodynamic compromise but with an EF of <35% should be offered an ICD. Other management options include EPS, checking, and correcting underlying causes, such as electrolyte disturbances, and antiarrhythmic medication.

Polymorphic VT

The most well-known form of polymorphic VT is torsade de pointes, which means 'turning on the points'. The axis moves from +ve to −ve (Fig. 12.5). The causes of this can be long QT syndrome, tricyclic antidepressants, bradycardia, and the effects of some antiarrhythmics. Treatment is aimed at establishing and treating the cause or, in some cases, overdrive pacing.

Catecholaminergic polymorphic VT

This is a genetic disorder where the QT interval may be either normal or short. It is often found in children or adolescents in the presence of exercise or stress. It can be treated with β-blockers or an ICD.

Long QT interval

This can be congenital (☐ Congenital long QT syndrome, p.287) or acquired. The QT interval is measured from the start of the QRS complex to the end of the T-wave. The QT interval varies with rate and ↑ as the heart rate ↓. It should be no more than half the length of the R–R interval. The Q–T interval ↑ with age and is longer in ♀.

SVT with aberrant conduction

In some instances, the impulse arrives through the AV node early while the His bundle and, in particular, the right bundle branch are still refractory. This can cause aberrant conduction. RBBB can usually be seen on the ECG. If the patient is tachycardic, it might be difficult to differentiate between SVT and VT. It is likely to be VT if the following signs are present:

• SVT with aberrant conduction is less common than VT.
• Left-axis deviation.

- Concordance in the chest leads (all complexes are in the same direction).
- QRS complex >0.14s.
- AV dissociation.
- No response to vagal manoeuvres.
- If the patient has a history of CHD or MI then it is more likely to be VT.
- It is better to always assume VT, unless proven otherwise.

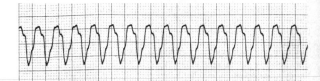

Fig. 12.4 Ventricular tachycardia.

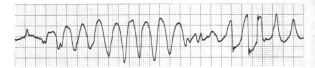

Fig. 12.5 Torsades de pointes.

[6] National Institute for Health and Clinical Excellence (2006) *Implantable Cardioverter Defibrillators for Arrhythmias*. NHS, London.

Ventricular fibrillation

VF (Fig. 12.6) is caused by chaotic activity in the ventricle, which leads to a cessation of cardiac contraction and cardiac arrest. It is life threatening and requires immediate treatment with CPR and defibrillation (📖 Advanced life support, p.341).

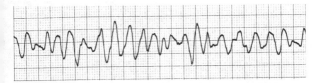

Fig. 12.6 Ventricular fibrillation.

Management of tachycardias

The management required depends on the individual patient and the advice of the clinician in charge of the patient's care. The suggested management for tachycardias is shown in Fig. 12.7.[7] In all cases of arrhythmia, the patient should be checked for adverse signs and symptoms and, if possible, an ECG should be performed. Adverse signs and symptoms include the following:

• Loss of pulse
• Loss of consciousness
• Chest pain
• Hypotension
• Heart failure.

Management of the arrhythmias can involve the following:
• Holter monitoring (used for diagnostic purposes)
• Correction of electrolytes such as potassium, calcium, and magnesium
• Vagal manoeuvres
• Treatment of adverse signs and symptoms as listed earlier.
• Electrical (e.g. antiarrhythmics) or DC cardioversion
• ICD insertion
• EPS and, in some cases, radiofrequency ablation (RFA).

If CSM is performed, warn the patient that it could make them feel dizzy; the patient should preferably be lying down while the procedure is carried out. If adenosine is administered, monitor the patient and warn them that they might experience an unpleasant sensation (adenosine can cause temporary asystole). The drug should be administered quickly and the nurse should also have atropine available in case a sustained, symptomatic bradycardia develops.

[7] Resuscitation Council (2010) *Advanced Life Support. Resuscitation* Council, London.

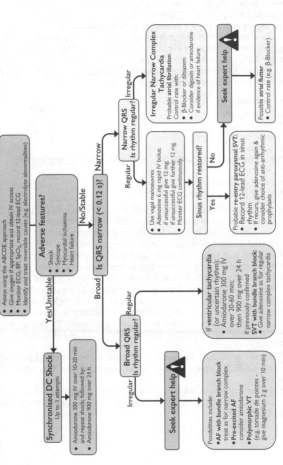

Fig. 12.7 Adult tachycardia (with pulse) algorithm. Used with kind permission by the Resuscitation Council (2010).

Direct current cardioversion

Cardioversion might be required for symptomatic SVT, atrial flutter, VT (with a pulse), and AF. Unlike defibrillation, the shock needs to be synchronized to coincide with the R-wave to prevent causing VF. The patient must be sedated or given a general anaesthetic because cardioversion can be very uncomfortable. It also must take place in a monitored environment. In some hospitals, it might occur in the CCU, ITU, A&E, HDU, or theatre. Cardioversion can be elective, i.e. for a chronic arrhythmia where drug therapy is either contraindicated or not tolerated, or may be urgent/emergency, i.e. in a peri-arrest situation.

Pre procedure
- Informed consent
- 12-lead ECG
- Bloods for electrolytes, INR, and digoxin levels
- IV access
- Attach the patient to cardiac monitoring, SpO$_2$ monitoring, and BP monitoring
- Baseline observations
- Remove patches and excessive chest hair.

The patient should be monitored throughout. The pads/paddles should be placed in the same position as for defibrillation (the anteroposterior position is more successful for AF). The synchronization button needs to be pressed before delivering a shock. On some machines, this must be done before each shock. It is important that the synchronization button is turned off after the procedure so that it does not interfere with defibrillation. There could be a delay between the button being pressed and the shock being delivered, which the operator must be aware of. If a biphasic machine is used, the machine should be set to 70–120J for SVT and atrial flutter or 120–150J for VT and AF. If this is not successful, deliver further shocks at higher J (refer to the manufacturer's guidelines). If a monophasic machine is used, set it at either 100J or 200J for SVT and atrial flutter or VT and AF, respectively.

After the procedure has been completed, monitor the patient and perform an ECG. Airway management is important until the patient is fully awake.

If the patient is at ↑ risk of a thromboembolic event, they should be anticoagulated for 1mth before and 1mth after cardioversion in case of emboli.

Implantable cardioverter-defibrillators

Ventricular tachyarrhythmias cause ~80% of SCD.[8] Although antiarrhythmics can help to suppress arrhythmias, they do not usually terminate them. Most ICDs consist of a pulse generator and electrodes, which can be in the right atria and ventricle or just the right ventricle. The power generator is usually positioned in the left pectoral area. An ICD can offer the following facilities:

• Monitor heart rate and rhythm, and record actions
• Antitachycardia pacing
• Pacing for bradycardia and post-shock pacing
• Cardioversion.
• Defibrillation
• Cardiac re-synchronization therapy (CRT).

The device will be programmed according to the individual needs of the patient.

Subcutaneous implantable defibrillators (S-ICD)

Newer S-ICDs have been developed. These do not contain any leads and will provide a shock of up to 80J when an arrhythmia is detected. The device is implanted into the skin under the left precordium. This may be performed under general or local anaesthetic. Two more incisions are made at the left side of the breastbone for electrodes to be inserted and attached to the generator. Although the S-ICD can provide transthoracic pacing post shock this is at a low rate and for a short period of time. It cannot provide antitachycardia pacing. Benefits of the S-ICD include the fact that it ↓ the risk of intracardiac infection associated with transvenous lead implantation.

NICE[8] recommends ICDs in the following situations:
• 1° prevention—for patients who have not had VT/VF but are at high risk:
  • History of previous MI (>4wks) and either an EF of <35% and nonsustained VT on a Holter monitor and VT on EPS or an EF of <30% and a QRS complex of =/> 0.12s.
  • A familial cardiac condition that has a high risk of SCD, such as HCM, long QT syndrome, Brugada syndrome, and ARVC.
• 2° prevention:
  • Patients who have survived a cardiac arrest resulting from VF/VT (in the absence of a treatable cause).
  • Spontaneous VT causing syncope or haemodynamic compromise.
  • Sustained VT without syncope or compromise but with an EF of <35%.

The preparation for ICD insertion is similar to that for a permanent pacemaker (□ Types of pacing, p.224). It is vital that the patient and family are given a lot of psychological support and that they fully understand the implications of the device. The ICD is inserted either under general anaesthetic or under a local anaesthetic with conscious sedation. After the leads have been inserted into the atria and ventricles the position is checked on an X-ray. The pulse generator is then inserted, and after the leads are attached, VT/VF is stimulated to test to see whether the ICD recognizes and terminates the arrhythmia.

After the procedure, monitor the patient initially. Observe the wound site for swelling, bleeding, and signs of infection. Arm movements must be limited for the first 24h. The patient might experience pain, so analgesia might be required. The patient can be discharged on the same day as the procedure or the following day. Before discharge, it is important that the patient and family are fully prepared for what might happen in the advent of an arrhythmia because this can cause some distress. The patient should be given an ID certificate and the number of their local centre for advice. There are a number of support groups that the patient could attend. Most activities can be resumed within 2–4wks, although they should avoid contact sports and situations that might be dangerous if they collapsed (e.g. climbing). ICD electrograms will be analysed at follow-up appointments to see what type of arrhythmia the patient is experiencing. Other advice is as follows:

- Carry and use a mobile phone away from the device.
- MRI scans over the insertion area are contraindicated.
- Microwave ovens are safe.
- Airport security alarms might be set off so carry the ID certificate.
- Record the date and time of any incidence and inform the local centre.
- Other people are not at risk of any shock.
- The patient might or might not lose consciousness during a shock or pacing.
- Some patients can experience warning symptoms before a shock.
- The battery life is up to 7yrs.
- Driving—no PSV or LGV licence. The patient can drive 1mth after the insertion if the ICD was implanted for VT without incapacity or if it is a prophylactic ICD insertion (see DVLA website for conditions). No driving for 6mths following ICD insertion associated with incapacity and then only if no shock or antitachycardia pacing. No driving for a month following revision of a device or alteration of antiarrhythmics. If box change only, driving can be resumed after 1wk.
- At some point there needs to be a discussion with the patient and family regarding switching the ICD off at the end of life. Some Trusts may have protocols regarding this.

The complications of ICD insertion include the following:

- Wound infection
- Migration of leads/device
- Inappropriate shocks
- Pneumothorax
- Haemothorax
- Embolism
- Lead dislodgement
- Bleeding.

---

[8] National Institute for Health and Clinical Excellence (2006) *Implantable Cardioverter Defibrillators for Arrhythmias*. NHS, London

Related guidance

European Society of Cardiology (2010) Guidelines for the management of atrial fibrillation. *European Heart Journal* **31**, 2369–429.

European Society of Cardiology (2012) Focused update of the ESC guidelines for management of atrial fibrillation. *European Heart Journal* **33**, 2719–47.

National Institute for Health and Clinical Excellence (2009) *Percutaneous (Non-thorascopic) Epicardial Catheter Radiofrequency Ablation for Atrial Fibrillation.* NICE, London.

National Institute for Health and Clinical Excellence (2009) *Thorascopic Epicardial Radiofrequency Ablation for Atrial Fibrillation.* NICE, London.

National Institute for Health and Clinical Excellence (2009) *Percutaneous (Non-thorascopic) Epicardial Catheter Radiofrequency Ablation for Ventricular Tachycardia.* NICE, London.

National Institute for Health and Clinical Excellence (2010) *Dronedarone for the Treatment of Non-permanent Atrial Fibrillation.* NICE, London.

National Institute for Health and Clinical Excellence (2010) *Percutaneous Occlusion of the Left Atrial Appendage in Non-valvular Atrial Fibrillation for the Prevention of Thromboembolism.* NICE, London.

National Institute for Health and Clinical Excellence (2011) *Thorascopic Exclusion of the Left Atrial Appendage (With or Without Surgical Ablation) for Non-valvular Atrial Fibrillation for the Prevention of Thromboembolism.* NICE, London.

National Institute for Health and Clinical Excellence(2011) *Percutaneous Endoscopic Catheter Laser Balloon Pulmonary Vein Isolation for Atrial Fibrillation.* NICE, London.

National Institute for Health and Clinical Excellence (2012) *Dabigatran Etexilate for the Prevention of Stroke and Systemic Embolism in Atrial Fibrillation.* NICE, London.

Related guidance

Electrophysiology

Introduction

This short chapter is intended for cardiac nurses who require a brief introduction to the highly complex specialty of cardiac electrophysiology (EP).

Further reading and case observation would be required to attain a firm understanding of the technical principles and applications of EP.

Much can be learned about a patient's cardiac rhythm from an ECG, e.g. AF, VT. However, more precise analysis is required to accurately define the origin and mechanism of an arrhythmia. The EP study (EPS) can help the physician make more informed decisions regarding arrhythmia therapy, which may include ablation.

Basic electrophysiology

- EP is the use of intracardiac electrograms (EGMs) to evaluate, diagnose, and potentially treat cardiac arrhythmias.
- EGMs are obtained by electrode catheters that are inserted into cardiac chambers and vessels.
- In contrast to an ECG, which records electrical activity of the entire heart, an EGM records only localized myocardial activation between two catheter electrodes. The displayed electrical signal coincides with the time that the wave of depolarization passes the catheter electrodes.
- If several electrode catheters are placed within the heart and EGMs are recorded at these various sites, the sequence of electrical activation throughout the heart can be observed (Fig. 13.1).

High right atrium (HRA) EGM

- The catheter is positioned in the superior portion of the RA as far from the ventricles as possible and as close to the SA node as possible.
- Displays EGM from HRA.

Coronary sinus (CS) EGM

- The catheter is positioned in the CS.
- EGMs are displayed from both the LA and the LV.

His bundle EGM

- The catheter is positioned over the septal aspect of the tricuspid valve, close to the His bundle and straddling the AV conduction system.
- A catheter placed in this position will record three separate and distinct EGMs.
- An EGM from the low RA is displayed.
- The His bundle EGM is displayed.
- An EGM from the RV is also displayed.

Right ventricular apex (RVA) EGM

The catheter is positioned in the apex of the RV and displays the RVA EGM. Note the ECG and corresponding EGMs in Fig. 13.1:

- The HRA EGM coincides with the P-wave onset.
- The atrial EGM on the His channel coincides nearer the end of the P-wave, and the RV EGM coincides with the QRS complex.
- Because electrical impulses conduct very quickly the waveforms are displayed at 100mm/s instead of the usual 25mm/s on a standard ECG. This effectively spreads the EGM signals out across the page. It enables more comprehensible observation of any change in activation sequence and greater accuracy in the measurement of basic intervals.
- The basic intervals of time are measured in ms (Fig. 13.1).

Basic cycle length (BCL)

The BCL is the time (in ms) between successive atrial EGMs and is also an indirect measure of HR. For example, if the BCL is 600ms, the HR can be calculated using the following formula:

$$60\ 000 \div BCL\ (ms) = HR\ (bpm)$$
$$60\ 000 \div 600ms = 100bpm$$

The number 60 000 is used in this simple formula because there are 60 000ms in 1min.

Atrial conduction (AC) time

The intra-atrial conduction time (IACT) or AC time is the time interval of electrical activity from the sinus node to the AV node. Measured from the surface P-wave onset to the atrial deflection on the His bundle EGM, it ranges from 25–55ms.

The atrium to His (AH) interval

This can be likened to the PR interval in an ECG but is more explicit. The AH interval is a measure of AV nodal conduction. It is measured between the low right atrial deflection and the His deflection on the His bundle EGM and ranges from 45–140ms.

The His to ventricle (HV) interval

The HV interval is a measure of intraventricular conduction. It is measured between the His deflection and the ventricular deflection on the His bundle EGM and ranges from 25–55ms.

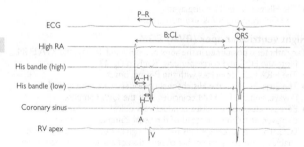

Fig. 13.1 Sweep speed 100mm/s. All measurements of ventricular activation line up under the QRS (between the two vertical lines on the second complex).

Electrophysiology catheters

The diagnostic EP catheter is made of electrically insulated wires attached to electrodes. The catheters are inserted into the blood vessels, usually through the femoral veins, and into the heart through the inferior vena cava. The electrodes are at the distal end of the catheter and are positioned by the physician to straddle the myocardial region of interest, e.g. the HRA, RVA, etc.

At the proximal end of the catheter the insulated wires are connected to a handle outside the patient which the doctor uses to manipulate the catheter. Cables attach the handle to a pacing stimulator and recording system. This arrangement enables the physician to monitor, measure, and record EGMs from the electrodes at the distal end of the catheter and to perform various pacing manoeuvres otherwise known as programmed electrical stimulation.

Electrophysiologists are able to place catheters with great precision. Some catheters have distal ends that can be steered by a mechanism in the handle. A tube, or sheath, is sometimes used to support and help guide the catheter to the desired location in the heart.

EP catheters are available in a variety of electrode configurations. Commonly used diagnostic catheters are quadrapolar (four electrodes) and decapolar (10 electrodes) catheters. Circular ring-like catheters with up to 20 electrodes may be used (Fig. 13.2). Each pair of electrodes makes a signal on the screen so a catheter with 10 electrodes displays five signals.

The ablation catheter is a special catheter in the electrophysiologist's arsenal as it is the only one that can deliver radiofrequency energy (Fig. 13.3). Some new ablation catheters allow the electrophysiologist to monitor the force being applied by the catheter to the walls of the heart chambers. This helps protect against perforation and is therefore safer for the patient but also helps the doctor to judge the effectiveness of each energy application.

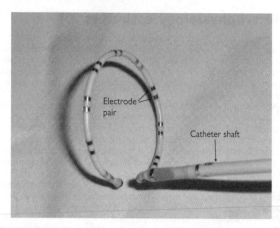

Fig. 13.2 Circular catheter for diagnostic evaluation of the pulmonary veins.

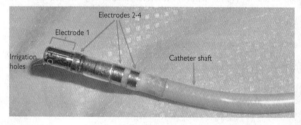

Fig. 13.3 Ablation catheter for delivering heat energy to the heart tissue.

Programmed electrical stimulation

- Pacing during the EPS is called programmed electrical stimulation (PES). Pacing is performed using two adjacent electrodes on a catheter. Any electrode pair can be used, even those on the ablation catheter.
- The EP catheter is connected to an external pacemaker or 'pacing stimulator'. An electrical current from the stimulator is delivered to an electrode on the EP catheter which may then depolarize the adjacent myocardium. This depolarization travels through the heart creating an artificially-generated heartbeat.
- PES is used to do four things:
  - assess the electrical behaviour of the heart at rest
  - initiate an arrhythmia (tachycardia)
  - assess electrical behaviour during tachycardia
  - terminate the tachycardia.
- These artificial (paced) beats closely mimic supraventricular ectopic beats (SVE) or ventricular ectopic beats (VE).
- In the human heart, a SVE or VE is often required to initiate a patient's arrhythmia. In the EP laboratory artificial (paced) SVEs or VEs do the same thing, initiating a patient's clinical tachycardia in a controlled clinical environment so it can then be analysed.
- The types of PES used are fixed pacing and extrastimulus pacing.

Fixed pacing

Fixed (also known as burst) pacing is a series of pacing impulses at stable cycle lengths. An example is pacing in the HRA (near the sinus node) at a fixed cycle length of 600ms. This would closely mimic sinus tachycardia at 100bpm.

60 000/600ms = 100bpm

During an EPS fixed pacing might last for a few beats, several minutes, or the entire duration of the case.

A variation of fixed pacing is incremental pacing where the rate of pacing is ↑ every few beats until a change in electrical conduction is seen.

Extrastimulus pacing

- Extrastimulus pacing involves adding extra pacing impulses at progressively shorter intervals following a short burst of fixed pacing.
- Here is an example: eight incremental pacing stimuli through the HRA catheter at 600ms (100bpm) plus one extrastimulus at 400ms (150bpm). The next extrastimulus might then be at 380ms.
- The extrastimulus technique often initiates the patient's tachycardia because the extra beats act like an artificial ectopic.
- More than one extrastimulus can be added which is said to be more 'aggressive' PES.

During PES the physician looks for changes in the pattern of electrical conduction on the EGM. The order of the depolarizations helps locate the extra electrical cells the tachycardia uses to sustain itself.

If tachycardia is induced the physician will examine the EGMs in various areas of the heart (like the CS and His). The EGMs may display a vastly different pattern during tachycardia compared to that of sinus rhythm. Initially it may be hard to tell what kind of tachycardia has been induced but luckily different tachycardias will respond to pacing manoeuvres in different ways. Pacing manoeuvres—pacing at different rates and from different parts of the heart—during tachycardia can further help to locate the extra pathway.

Just as a tachycardia can be induced by PES it can also be terminated by pacing. If the patient is haemodynamically unstable (i.e. low BP) due to the induced tachycardia—and pacing does not terminate tachycardia—the patient may require cardioversion.

Once the location of the extra cells is established the physician can then ablate them and stop the tachycardia from occurring.

Ablation

When the PES is complete and the local myocardial region supporting the clinical tachycardia has been identified by examination of the EGMs, the tachycardia can be permanently terminated by delivering energy through a special ablation catheter. Ablation is the application of energy to the myocardium to modify and essentially obliterate its electrical excitability. The effect on the tissue is permanent.

By far the most widely used form of energy delivery is radiofrequency ablation (RFA). RF energy is a low-voltage electrical current. The application of RF energy to the myocardium creates lesions at the site of delivery. The tip of an RF ablation catheter is commonly 4mm long and 2mm in diameter which creates lesions roughly 5mm in diameter and 3mm in depth. Stable contact during the RF application is important to sufficiently treat the myocardium. Effective application times vary from a few seconds up to a minute (and sometimes longer) for adequate treatment depending on the site of ablation and the type of arrhythmia being treated. Deeper (thicker) tissue such as LV myocardium may require longer applications of ablation.

The abnormal tissue can also be treated using cryoablation whereby the tissue is altered by freezing. The cryoablation catheter is connected to a refrigeration console, which creates cryogenic temperatures at the tip of the catheter. A temperature of −70°C is required for permanent ablation. Precise mapping of the critical ablation site can be performed by temporarily chilling the region to only −30°C. The tissue can only be temporarily modified at this temperature. This might be of benefit where ablation is required to treat tachycardias that arise nearby high-risk sites like the AV node. The potential ablation site can be tested without permanent obliteration of this crucial structure. If the arrhythmia is successfully treated at this lower temperature without damaging the AV node, permanent cryoablation can be performed at −70°C.

Tachycardias that can be ablated include atrial flutter, atrioventricular nodal re-entrant tachycardia (AVNRT), atrioventricular re-entrant tachycardia (AVRT), atrial tachycardia, and ventricular tachycardia.

Ablation can be used to treat AF. These procedures may take up to 5h and success rates are lower than for most other supraventricular arrhythmias. Repeat procedures may be required. Many patients are not suitable for this kind of procedure and are instead treated with medications. Paroxysmal AF ablation has a higher success rate than persistent AF.

AF ablation is performed in the LA as this is the chamber where the arrhythmia actively occurs. The RA does contract during AF but this occurs passively and it is not directly involved in the arrhythmia.

AF ablation is performed in the LA as this is the chamber where the arrhythmia actively occurs. The RA does contract during AF but this occurs passively and it is not directly involved in the arrhythmia.

The pulmonary veins play an important role in causing AF so disconnecting them electrically from the rest of the LA is a major part of any AF procedure. Most doctors begin by using the ablation catheter to draw a continuous ring of lesions around the right and left pulmonary veins (PVs). Ectopic beats from the veins that can initiate AF no longer conduct into the atrium. The physician may encircle all four veins separately or both left veins and both right veins as pairs. This is usually enough for ablation of PAF. This procedure may be called pulmonary vein isolation (PVI), left atrial circumferential ablation (LACA), or wide area circumferential ablation (WACA).

For persistent AF more extensive ablation is required. After PVI is performed ablation energy may be delivered at sites where special EGMs called complex fractionated atrial electrograms (CFAEs) are seen. Burning these CFAEs, which are thought to be major contributors to AF, helps to treat this arrhythmia. Straight lines of lesions may also be used which can cause further disruption to the electrical conduction of AF. Common linear lesions are 'roof lines' and 'mitral isthmus lines' which join electrically inert structures to each other. The lines act like an impassable wall to electrical conduction.

Ablation of atrial tachycardia (AT) is also possible. These arrhythmias can be focal or macro-re-entrant. The origin of a focal AT can be pin-pointed in the lab using mapping techniques. Energy can then be applied to ablate this small region of tissue stopping the tachycardia and preventing it from restarting.

Macro-re-entrant AT is a continuous wavefront of depolarization going around and around a large part of either atrium. Mapping and pacing techniques help to establish the path taken by the tachycardia. The path is then cut by linear ablation lesions. Just as in AF, the lesions act like a wall that the wavefront cannot get past and the tachycardia is stopped.

Typical (or isthmus-dependent) atrial flutter is a common type of macro-re-entrant AT that takes a set path in the RA. This is relatively easy to ablate compared to AF and most ATs by creating a linear lesion from the tricuspid annulus to the inferior vena cavae. This is known as a 'line of block'.

While most ablation procedures are not urgent, VT is a life-threatening rhythm which is sometimes best treated with ablation. Various type of mapping may be employed including pace mapping, voltage mapping (which helps to find scarred tissue from myocardial infarction), and activation mapping (which looks at the timing of signals). The electrophysiologist decides which mapping techniques to use depending on how haemodynamically stable the patient is during VT and for how long, and how often, the patient is in VT.

EPS and ablations may be performed under conscious sedation or general anaesthetic.

Nursing considerations

The principles of nursing care for patients undergoing EPS/RFA and coronary angiography are very similar. In addition to the care for a patient before and after angiography (⌨ Coronary angiography: preprocedure care, p.139; Coronary angiography: postprocedure care, p.142), the patient undergoing EPS/RFA requires the following:

Pre procedure

Discuss with the patient the purpose of the procedure, which is to induce the arrhythmia. This enables the electrophysiologist to gather as much information about the arrhythmia as possible and tailor treatment to the individual needs of the patient. It is, ∴, essential to perform a thorough assessment of the patient and their symptoms before the procedure, in particular the occurrence of syncope. The patient is likely to experience these symptoms during the procedure and must be prepared for this. It is also important to reassure the patient that equipment and medication is available to terminate the arrhythmia.

In some cases, antiarrhythmic medications might be discontinued before the procedure; ∴, careful observation of the patient's heart rhythm is essential.

During procedure

Drugs such as isoprenaline, atropine, and adenosine may be used to help define the location of extra electrical pathways by temporarily altering the electrical characteristics of the heart. During left atrial and ventricular procedures heparin is used to avoid stroke by inhibiting thrombus formation around the catheters.

Post procedure

Again, the purpose of frequent observations is to detect procedural complications. In addition to those described following angiography (⌨ Coronary angiography: postprocedure care, p.142), it is important to observe for cardiac tamponade following transseptal puncture and arrhythmias (⌨ Cardiac tamponade, p.347). Nurses who care for patients with arrhythmias should be prepared to handle any emergency that might arise. Following successful ablation, antiarrhythmic medications are usually discontinued. Following AF ablation, patients usually continue taking warfarin.

Related guidance

Chen HS, Wen JM, Wu SN, Lui JP (2012) *Catheter Ablation for Paroxysmal and Persistent AF.* *Cochrane Database of Systematic Reviews* **4**, CD007101. doi: 10.1002/14651858.CD007101.pub2.

National Institute for Health and Clinical Excellence (2009) *Percutaneous (Non-Thoracoscopic) Epicardial Catheter Radio-Frequency Ablation for Atrial Fibrillation.* NICE, London.

National Institute for Health and Clinical Excellence (2009) *Percutaneous (Non-Thoracoscopic) Epicardial Catheter Radio-Frequency Ablation for Ventricular Tachycardia.* NICE, London.

Congenital heart disease and inherited cardiac disorders

Introduction

'Congenital heart disease' is a term used to cover a wide range of cardiac conditions that result from an abnormality of cardiac structure or function present at birth. Most conditions are a result of the heart, its valves, or its vessels not being properly formed. Some congenital heart defects are diagnosed *in utero* or soon after birth, whereas others might not be noted until later in life when symptoms become troublesome. Defects can be simple (requiring little or no intervention), moderate (requiring episodic intervention), or complex (with serious outcomes that require life-long treatment and follow-up).

The majority of children with congenital heart disease are managed in specialist paediatric centres, and as more children with congenital heart disease survive into adulthood, services that cater for adults with congenital heart disease (ACHD) have been developed. Most cardiac nurses working in the cardiac arena can be expected to care for adult patients with congenital heart disease at some time in their career. They might also care for patients who present for the first time in adulthood with inherited disorders that have significant cardiovascular problems. The focus of this chapter is to highlight some of the issues that ACHD patients might present with in cardiac areas that do not specialize in ACHD. It is outside the scope of this chapter to provide detailed coverage of cardiac embryology and the development of the heart *in utero*. It is also not possible to cover the range of corrective surgery, palliative surgery, percutaneous procedures, and the specialist management of congenital heart disease that many of this patient group will have undergone in the past. This chapter covers the following topics:

- An overview of the development of services for ACHD.
- A brief outline of the fetal circulation.
- A basic outline of common congenital heart defects.
- A basic outline of common inherited disorders that have associated cardiac problems.
- The common signs and symptoms that patients might present with as adults.
- Nursing considerations.

Cardiomyopathy is covered separately in Chapter 15.

Adults with congenital heart disease

Major advances in the treatment of congenital heart disease within the past 20yrs mean that many more neonates and children with congenital heart problems survive into adulthood. Children born in the 1960s had a 10% 18yr survival rate, but this has ↑ to 50% in the 1980s, requiring the development of services for ACHD (also known as 'grown-ups with congenital heart disease' [GUCH]). Because the number of ACHD patients will continue to ↑ in years to come, these services are expected to continue to expand. A hub and spoke model of care is recommended with specialist centres in the middle but with a continued process of two-way communication between the specialist centre and other providers of care such as the patient's local hospital.[1] Shared care should be multidisciplinary, with specialties such as dentistry, obstetrics, and anaesthetics developing relevant expertise. Routine monitoring of anticoagulation, cardiac medication, and blood chemistry may be managed by 1° care staff. Many patients with congenital heart disease also have learning disabilities and healthcare staff must be mindful of the special needs of this patient group. It is envisaged that many protocols for shared care will be developed in the future, and it is imperative that cardiac nurses are familiar with these and know how to access specialist advice, as necessary.

[1] Department of Health (2006) *Adult Congenital Heart Disease: A Commissioning Guide for Services for Young People and Grown Ups with Congenital Heart Disease (GUCH)*. DH, London.

Fetal circulation

The cardiovascular system evolves into a highly specialized four-chamber heart with associated vasculature by following a set sequence of complex events. Any interruption in this sequence or abnormal development can result in congenital heart defects.

The developing embryo has a high demand for oxygen because of the proliferating tissue. Because blood bypasses the developing lungs in the embryo, it receives blood oxygenated at the placenta (in the capillaries of the chorionic villi) through a single umbilical vein (see Fig. 14.1). In the fetal circulation, blood moves from the right side of the heart to the left side through the foramen ovale, bypassing the RV. Additionally, the ductus arteriosus ensures that most blood from the pulmonary artery flows into the aorta, yet also allows sufficient blood to be supplied to the developing lung tissue. The ductus venosus enables most of the oxygenated blood to bypass the liver. Deoxygenated blood is returned to the placenta via the umbilical arteries (see Fig. 14.1).

At birth, three main events occur, as follows:
• Pulmonary gas exchange: disruption of placental blood flow triggers inspiration, lung inflation, and subsequent pulmonary blood flow.
• Foramen ovale closure: ↑ LA pressure closes the foramen ovale.
• The ductus arteriosus, umbilical arteries, and ductus venosus close soon after birth.

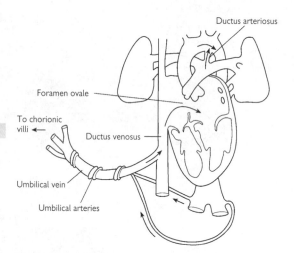

Fig. 14.1 The fetal circulation before birth. Adapted with permission from Chikwe J, Beddow E, and Glenville B (2006). *Cardiothoracic Surgery*. Oxford University Press, Oxford.

Classification of congenital heart disease

Congenital heart disease in adults is generally divided into two main sub-types: acyanotic and cyanotic lesions. This division relates to whether cyanosis is a predominant presenting symptom. The common defects are listed in Table 14.1.

Table 14.1 Classification of congenital heart defects

Acyanotic	Cyanotic
• Atrial septal defect (ASD)	• Transposition of the great arteries (TGA)
• Ventricular septal defect (VSD)	• Tetralogy of Fallot (TOF)
• Pulmonary stenosis (PS)	
• Coarctation of the aorta (COA)	
• Patent ductus arteriosus (PDA)	

Septal defects

Both ASDs and VSDs are commonly called 'holes in the heart'. ASDs and VSDs may occur in isolation or may occur with other defects such as TOF.

Atrial septal defect

This is the most common defect in adults after bicuspid aortic valve. An ASD is an opening or communication between left and right atria, with midseptal defects occurring most frequently. There are four types: ostium secundum (most common), sinus venosus, ostium primum, and coronary sinus defects.

ASD repair usually occurs in childhood. Small ASDs might, however, go undetected in childhood and may only be detected in adulthood when the patient is having medical treatment for something else or may be picked up during pregnancy. Adults with untreated ASDs might present with gradually worsening symptoms in their 40s onwards. Initially the patient will have a shunt of blood from the left ventricle to the right; however this shunt may be temporarily reversed during Valsalva type manoeuvres such as coughing and straining. This can lead to a TIA or even stroke. Long term the shunt may cause overload and dilatation of the RA and RV which can lead to arrhythmias and other problems such as heart failure, pulmonary ↑ BP and ↓ exercise capacity.

Signs and symptoms
- SOBOE
- Recurrent chest infection
- ↓ exercise tolerance.
- Atrial arrhythmias, such as AF
- Palpitations.

Investigations
- CXR—cardiomegaly may be present
- ECG—AF, evidence of atrial hypertrophy
- Cardiac catheter—useful if ↑ PAP on Echo to establish PVR
- TOE

Management
If a significant shunt has developed the ASD should be closed regardless of symptoms to prevent further problems. Secundum defects are the only type that can be closed using a percutaneous device. The majority of secundum defects can be done in this way if the defect is <4cm diameter. The patient may only require an overnight stay and may be on antiplatelet therapy for 3–6mths.

Other types of ASDs and larger secundum defects require surgical closure (see Chapter 9).

Patent foramen ovale

A PFO is a remnant of normal fetal circulation rather than a true ASD and is present in up to 30% of the population. However, it can be clinically significant because the first indication of a PFO can be an unexplained stroke (CVA). It may also be associated with migraine with aura. There may not be any signs or symptoms and it may also not show any abnormalities on ECG, CXR, or Echo. Indications for closure include embolic stroke. It can also be done for recurrent migraine however this would only be for those severely affected by recurrent, refractory migraine that have been carefully selected by a neurologist and interventional cardiologist. Closure is usually by deploying a percutaneous closure device.

Ventricular septal defect

This is the most common defect found in children, but ~70% of VSDs close spontaneously. A VSD is an opening between left and right ventricles. If significant, left-to-right shunting is present (whereby oxygenated blood is shunted back into the RV); the defect is usually surgically closed in childhood. Left untreated it can lead to CCF, ↑ PVR and ↑ risk of IE. Adults with small, persistent VSDs require regular follow-up. Some might present with IE later in life. VSD can also be the result of MI or trauma. VSDs may be closed surgically or percutaneously depending on the size and location of the VSD. Complications of repair include aortic valve regurgitation and heart blocks.

Untreated left-to-right shunts such as those in septal defects can result in the development of Eisenmenger syndrome (☐ Eisenmenger syndrome, p.285).

Right ventricular outflow tract obstructions

Pulmonary stenosis

This is commonly congenital in origin and can be valvular, subvalvular, or supravalvular. It is often associated with other defects, such as an ASD or VSD. In valvular stenosis, the valve leaflets are thickened and abnormal. PS causes obstruction of the RVOT and subsequent high RV pressures, which can lead to a right-to-left shunt. Some children with severe PS rely on a PDA to maintain adequate oxygenation. Severe PS requires treatment, which is usually in the form of balloon valvoplasty; although in some cases surgical valvotomy is required (see also 📖 Pulmonary valve disorders, p.89)

Pulmonary arterial hypertension (PAH)

PAH is defined as an elevated mean PAP >25mmHg with a pulmonary capillary wedge pressure <15mmHg. While not strictly just a congenital condition it has been included here as it may often be associated with other congenital conditions. It is a progressive condition that leads to right heart failure. It falls into group one of the World Health Organization classification of pulmonary hypertension:

* Group 1—pulmonary arterial hypertension:
  * idiopathic, familial, associated with other diseases such as HIV infection, congenital defects, venous or capillary disease
* Group 2—pulmonary hypertension associated with left heart disease:
  * atrial or ventricular disease; valve disease
* Group 3—pulmonary hypertension associated with lung diseases and/ or hypoxemia:
  * COPD; chronic exposure to high altitude
* Group 4—pulmonary hypertension due to chronic thrombotic and/or embolic disease:
  * PE; embolization of other matter
* Group 5—miscellaneous.

It mainly affects ♀ and may not be diagnosed until later life depending on the cause.

Signs and symptoms include:
* Dyspnoea on exertion
* Fatigue
* Chest pain
* Dizziness and syncope
* Cough
* Peripheral oedema and abdominal distension may be present when RVF develops.

Investigations:
* Echo
* ECG—RAH, RVH, RBBB
* CXR
* Lung function tests
* Right heart catheterization.

Management

Management of PAH is aimed at reducing symptoms, improving functional capacity, preventing disease progression, and ↓ mortality. Treatment may include O_2 therapy, diuretics, calcium-channel antagonists, and other vasodilators.

Patients should be encouraged to be active within the limits of their symptoms and some may be able to participate in tailored rehabilitation. Counselling and psychological support are very important. Pregnancy is contraindicated due to the ↑ mortality rate.

Other acyanotic lesions

Coarctation of the aorta

COA is the narrowing of the aorta, commonly just below the origin of the left subclavian artery. It is usually diagnosed in infancy and is surgically corrected. Occasionally, in less severe cases, it might not be diagnosed until adulthood. The patient usually has weak or absent femoral pulse. It is often associated with a congenital bicuspid aortic valve. COA requires surgical or percutaneous intervention. Adults might present with re-coarctation after previous surgical intervention. Hypertension is common and should be treated pharmacologically.

Patent ductus arteriosus

The ductus arteriosus should close shortly after birth. Most patients with a PDA will have had corrective surgery in childhood. Adults with a persistent small lumen ductus arteriosus might be discovered in later life, but are usually asymptomatic. Discovery of a moderate or large PDA in adults is rare.

Cyanotic lesions

Transposition of the great arteries

In this congenital defect, the aorta arises from the RV and the pulmonary artery arises from the LV. Consequently, the systemic and pulmonary circulatory systems are separate, and unless there is some other anomaly creating a link between the two systems, life is not sustainable. Most babies born with TGA also have one of the following:

- PFO
- ASD
- VSD
- PDA.

The coexistence of these lesions allows some mixing of blood and various degrees of oxygenated blood to reach the tissues, but despite this, the baby becomes profoundly cyanosed. Surgical intervention is mandatory.

There is also a congenitally corrected TGA, in which the baby is born with transposed ventricles, in addition to transposed great arteries. Thus, a semblance of a normal circulation is sustained. Most cases are detected in childhood, but it might go unnoticed until adulthood, when arrhythmias are common.

Tetralogy of Fallot

This can present with various abnormalities, but typically TOF has four lesions, as follows (see Fig. 14.2):

- PS
- Overriding aorta
- VSD
- RVH.

These anomalies result in a right-to-left shunt. Cyanosis develops as systemic deoxygenated venous blood mixes with oxygenated pulmonary venous blood. Surgical intervention is almost always required in early childhood and depends on the severity of the abnormalities. Previously, initial palliative surgery was performed before later corrective surgery. Today, babies born with TOF can undergo corrective surgery in infancy.

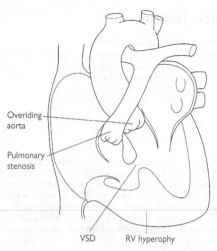

Overiding aorta

Pulmonary stenosis

VSD   RV hyperophy

Fig. 14.2 Tetralogy of Fallot. Adapted with permission from Chikwe J, Beddow E, and Glenville B (2006). *Cardiothoracic Surgery*. Oxford University Press, Oxford.

Eisenmenger syndrome

Eisenmenger syndrome occurs as a result of ↑ pulmonary vascular resistance, permanent pulmonary hypertension, and a consequent reverse shunt developing. The condition is progressive and irreversible; progression of Eisenmenger syndrome is slow, but it can result in premature death. Treatment is symptomatic or with a heart–lung transplant. Pregnancy in those with Eisenmenger syndrome is not advised because of the high maternal and fetal mortality rates.

Inherited cardiac syndromes presenting in later life

In addition to the congenital heart defects already noted, there are some inherited syndromes that might not be discovered until adulthood but have significant cardiac complications. These syndromes are outlined as follows:

Marfan's syndrome

This is a disorder of connective tissue, which has the following abnormalities:

- Skeletal: patients are tall, with long limbs and fingers. They might have scoliosis or chest-wall deformities. Patients usually have a high, arched palate.
- Eye: dislocation of the lens, myopia, retinal detachment, and glaucoma.
- Respiratory: pneumothorax, emphysema, and bronchiectasis.
- Cardiovascular: aortic root dilatation, AR, MVP, and MR.

Marfan's syndrome is an autosomal-dominant genetic disorder, i.e. it affects ♂ and ♀ equally, with only one copy of the gene required to cause the disorder. Moreover, if the gene is not inherited, the syndrome cannot be passed on. In one-quarter of cases, it is caused by a new genetic mutation, whereby the patient develops the syndrome without inheriting it. Patients can present with a variety of symptoms; it is estimated that ~10% of those affected will have serious health problems.

Nurses might care for patients with either established or newly diagnosed Marfan's syndrome, and patients will require support appropriate to their symptoms and how recently they have been diagnosed. Cardiac abnormalities associated with Marfan's syndrome usually require surgical intervention. Those diagnosed with Marfan's syndrome, but who do not have cardiac anomalies, require regular follow-up and echocardiography for early detection of cardiac abnormalities.

Brugada syndrome

This is an inherited disease that is caused by a mutation of a cardiac sodium-channel gene. It is an autosomal-dominant genetic disorder, affecting 3 in 1000 people in the Western world. The prevalence in Asia is thought to be much higher, although the reason for this disparity in prevalence is unknown.

Brugada syndrome is characterized by episodes of rapid polymorphic VT in which the patient has either a syncopal attack or a cardiac arrest if it degenerates into VF. It is most common in those in those aged 30–50yrs, but can occur at any age. A patient with this syndrome probably has a history of syncope or cardiac arrests; however, there are often no warning symptoms and the patient might die in their sleep.

In those with Brugada syndrome who survive, the ECG shows one of three distinctive patterns that are similar to complete or incomplete RBBB (see Fig. 14.3)

- Type 1: prominent coved ST-segment elevation in V1–V3, followed by a negative T-wave.
- Type 2: high ST-segment take-off and elevation, followed by a positive T-wave with saddleback configuration.
- Type 3: ST-segment elevation in V1–V3, which might be saddleback or coved, or both.

The treatment of choice for those with diagnosed or highly suspected Brugada syndrome is usually insertion of an ICD. Diagnosis is inherently difficult, but any patient with a history of unexplained syncope and a family history of sudden death at a young age should be referred to an electrophysiologist.

Congenital long QT syndrome

Long QT syndrome can be inherited or acquired (Ventricular tachycardia, p.251). Congenital long QT syndrome is an autosomal-dominant disorder associated with SCD. It is caused by mutations in at least five genes, all of which modulate the function of sodium or potassium ion channels. The abnormal ion channels prolong the repolarization process and the QT interval is >0.46s. This results in polymorphic VT or torsades des pointes, which often resembles VF (Ventricular tachycardia, p.251). This chaotic rhythm causes syncope or sudden unexpected death. The symptoms are triggered by different things according to the gene affected, including swimming and diving, exercise, loud noises, or sleep.

▶ After one family member is diagnosed with long QT syndrome, it is imperative that all family members are examined and referred to an electrophysiologist. Specialist advice and counselling are required for families who have a history of either Brugada syndrome or long QT syndrome, because if one person within a family has either syndrome, there is a high probability that others within the family will also be affected.

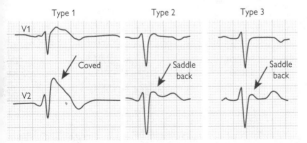

Fig. 14.3 ECG traces characteristic of Brugada syndrome. Adapted with permission from Firman E (2006). Diagnosing and treating Brugada syndrome. *Brit J Cardiac Nurs*, 1:7, pp. 332–7 © MA Healthcare.

Problems associated with congenital heart disease in adulthood

As previously stated, most ACHD patients with complex abnormalities and persistent cardiac problems receive specialist follow-up. However, many patients who have had previously corrected or undetected congenital defects might also be admitted to a general cardiac unit. The most common problems that they could present with are as follows:

- Arrhythmias: both atrial and ventricular arrhythmias can lead to significant haemodynamic deterioration, which is poorly tolerated in ACHD patients.
- Heart failure: caused by ↑ ventricular workload.
- IE: most ACHD patients have a life-long risk of IE, and nonspecific symptoms of malaise or persistent pyrexia should not be ignored in this group of patients. Acne in younger adults can be a source of IE. Body piercing or tattoos can also pose a risk. Prophylactic antibiotics are no longer recommended unless the patient is undergoing a high-risk procedure and has a high-risk condition (see Chapter 5, 📖 Patient education, p.107).
- Syncope: syncope in any ACHD patient must be investigated because it could be caused by arrhythmias or severe obstruction to the LVOT.
- Polycythaemia: chronic hypoxaemia leads to a compensatory ↑ in red blood cells and haemoglobin, which can lead to an ↑ in blood viscosity and resultant symptoms of headache, impaired alertness, muscle weakness, paraesthesia, or embolic events, such as stroke. These patients require haemodilution, whereby a controlled amount of blood is removed (usually 500mL) and replaced with glucose or saline. This can cause iron deficiency and, ∴, patients should take iron supplements.
- Surgery: either palliative or corrective surgery might be required in later life, usually because of restenosis, regurgitation, or conduit obstruction. Surgery should be carried out by a specialist surgeon.

Nursing considerations

Nursing considerations should be related to the symptoms of the patient, and careful haemodynamic monitoring is imperative because slight deterioration can be poorly tolerated. However, there are additional factors that nurses must consider for ACHD patients, especially younger adults who might be making health and lifestyle decisions that could be significantly affected by their condition.

Specialist referral

There are specialist services for ACHD and these are always available for advice and referral, as necessary. It is advisable for nurses to be aware of the contact information for their nearest ACHD centre. However, note that ACHD patients often have a wealth of specialist knowledge themselves and will have contact details for their own specialist.

Psychological support

ACHD patients face very real challenges in their lives not only in terms of their physical health, but also in terms of their lifestyle. ACHD patients might have difficulties in gaining employment or insurance or obtaining mortgages. This obviously depends on the severity of their cardiac problems and many lead full and active lives. However, recurrence of physical ill-health problems can trigger anger, stress, or depression in relation to their financial, employment, and social status. Nurses must give appropriate psychological support in relation to their patient's particular needs.

Health advice

Advice in relation to travel, contraception, pregnancy, and unrelated medical care should be given by specialist healthcare professionals. It is important to reinforce advice in the following areas:

- Travel advice: patients with cyanosis need to arrange supplemental O_2 for long-haul flights and require extra hydration. Travel insurance might be difficult to obtain, but some specialist insurance companies will provide it.
- Contraception: women with polycythaemia should not use the combined contraceptive pill because of an ↑ risk of thrombosis. Intrauterine coils can carry a risk of infection on insertion and, ∴, antibiotic prophylaxis is advised.
- Pregnancy: pre-pregnancy counselling is advisable for all ACHD patients because the risks and outcomes of pregnancy are dependent on the particular cardiac defect. All ACHD patients should have full medical and genetic assessments before considering pregnancy (📖 Heart disease in pregnancy, p.320).
- Noncardiac surgery: ACHD patients should be advised that noncardiac surgery and diagnostic procedures should be undertaken in specialist centres or with specialist advice regarding anaesthetic and infection risks.

Related guidance

Baumgartner H, Bonhoeffer P, De Groot N, et al. (2010) ESC Guidelines for the management of grown-up congenital heart disease. *European Heart Journal* **31**, 2915–57.

Galie N, Hoeper M, Humbert M, et al. (2009) Guidelines for the diagnosis and treatment of pulmonary hypertension. *European Heart Journal* **30**, 2493–537.

National Institute for Health and Clinical Excellence (2007) *Percutaneous Pulmonary Valve Implantation for Right Ventricular Outflow Tract Dysfunction*. NICE, London.

National Institute for Health and Clinical Excellence (2010) *Transcatheter Endovascular Closure of Perimembranous Ventricular Septal Defect*. NICE, London.

National Institute for Health and Clinical Excellence (2010) *Percutaneous Closure of Patent Foramen Ovale for Recurrent Migraine*. NICE, London.

Cardiomyopathy

Introduction

Cardiomyopathy is a descriptive term that means 'disease of the heart muscle': 'cardia' refers to the heart and 'myopathy' literally means an abnormality of muscle.

Cardiomyopathies are disorders of the myocardium that are not 2° to coronary artery disease, hypertension, congenital, valvular, or pericardial abnormalities. Cardiomyopathy is associated with myocardial dysfunction and is classified into the following four major subtypes

- Hypertrophic
- Dilated
- Arrhythmogenic right ventricular
- Restrictive.

The aim of this chapter is to outline the background, clinical presentation, diagnosis, treatment, and the role of the nurse in the management of the cardiomyopathies.

Hypertrophic cardiomyopathy (HCM): overview

HCM affects ~1 in 500 of the general population; it affects ♂ and ♀ in equal proportions and occurs in all ethnic groups. HCM can be idiopathic, but it is generally a genetically inherited disorder and has an autosomal-dominant pattern of inheritance. Each child independently has a 50% chance of inheriting the gene. Not all gene positive individuals develop the disease—a phenomenon known as incomplete penetrance. In some families, penetrance appears complete (Fig. 15.1), in others generational 'skips' may appear (Fig. 15.7).

A gene mutation can be identified in 50–60% of HCM patients. Several hundred mutations affecting >10 genes (most are sarcomeric genes) have been identified as causes. Manifestation of the disease within families can vary considerably, in that some family members can have a much milder form of the disease than other individuals within the family.

HCM is characterized by myocardial hypertrophy (thickened heart muscle), which can affect the left and/or the right ventricle. Most commonly, hypertrophy occurs in the interventricular septum, causing asymmetric septal hypertrophy (ASH; Fig. 15.2). Muscle thickening might be evenly distributed throughout the ventricle (symmetric/concentric left ventricular hypertrophy; Fig. 15.3) or concentrated at the apex of the heart (Fig. 15.4). HCM is also characterized by myocyte disarray and fibrosis, in which the cardiac muscles cells are misaligned and disorganized and can be irregular in shape and enlarged compared with normal myocytes. These characteristics probably contribute to the diastolic dysfunction and arrhythmias that patients with HCM are known to experience.

In some patients with ASH, obstruction of the flow of blood from the ventricle to the aorta can occur. The muscle thickening may be such that during systole the enlarged interventricular septum and the mitral valve press against one another, significantly narrowing the LVOT and thus obstructing the flow of blood out into the aorta (Fig. 15.5).

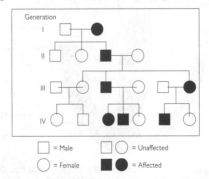

Fig. 15.1 Family tree showing four generations affected by hypertrophic cardiomyopathy. With kind permission from the Cardiomyopathy Association ℛ http://www.cardiomyopathy.org.

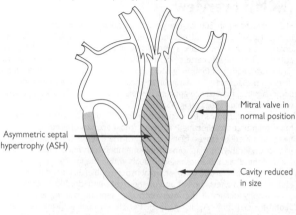

Fig. 15.2 Asymmetric septal hypertrophy. With kind permission from the Cardiomyopathy Association ✍ http://www.cardiomyopathy.org.

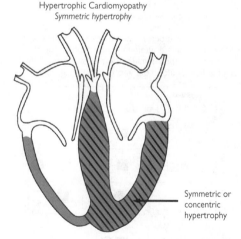

Fig. 15.3 Symmetric septal hypertrophy. With kind permission from the Cardiomyopathy Association ✍ http://www.cardiomyopathy.org.

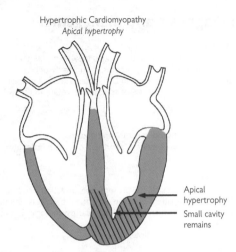

Hypertrophic Cardiomyopathy
Apical hypertrophy

Apical
hypertrophy

Small cavity
remains

Fig. 15.4 Apical hypertrophy. With kind permission from the Cardiomyopathy Association ℘ http://www.cardiomyopathy.org.

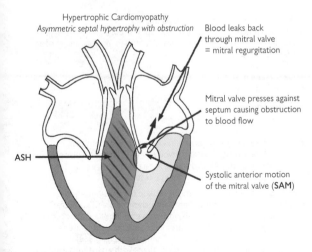

Hypertrophic Cardiomyopathy
Asymmetric septal hypertrophy with obstruction

Blood leaks back
through mitral valve
= mitral regurgitation

Mitral valve presses against
septum causing obstruction
to blood flow

ASH

Systolic anterior motion
of the mitral valve (**SAM**)

Fig. 15.5 Asymmetric septal hypertrophy with obstruction. With kind permission from the Cardiomyopathy Association ℘ http://www.cardiomyopathy.org.

HCM: diagnosis and management

Clinical presentation

Patients with HCM can present at any age; they might be asymptomatic or might experience only mild symptoms, including dyspnoea, chest pain, palpitations/arrhythmias, syncope, and, in some cases, SCD, which occurs in up to 1% of adults and up to 4% of adolescents/young adults with HCM (see Box 15.1).

History

- Family history (e.g. of sudden death) and pedigree.
- Symptoms—chest pain, dizziness, shortness of breath, palpitations, syncope.

Investigations

Depending on the patient's clinical presentation, investigations can be performed either on an in-patient or on an out-patient basis. It is vital that the nurse ensures that the patient is physically and psychologically prepared for any investigations.

Investigations include the following:

- 12-lead ECG
- TTE (□ Imaging studies: echocardiography, p.74)
- Family screening—detailed patient and family histories
- EPS (□ Basic electrophysiology, p.263)
- Holter or ambulatory monitoring (□ Ambulatory monitoring, p.72).

Other possible investigations are as follows:

- Angiography (□ Coronary angiography: preprocedure care, p.139)
- Advanced cardiac imaging (□ Imaging studies: nuclear and cardiac magnetic resonance, p.76)
- ETT (□ Exercise tolerance testing, p.71)
- CXR (□ Chest X-ray (CXR), p.64)
- Genetic testing.

Management

Management seeks to:

- Confirm diagnosis
- Establish symptom status and individualize treatment plan
- Establish prognostic risk and involvement from ventricular arrhythmias and sudden death, AF and stroke, heart failure
- Initiate family screening and genetic testing.

Pharmacological treatments might include the following:

- β-blockers—useful for patients with chest pain and particularly advantageous for those with obstructive HCM (□ β-blockers, p.366).
- Calcium-channel blockers—useful for patients with chest pain and obstructive HCM (□ Calcium-channel blockers, p.368).
- Antiarrhythmic medication—for patients with arrhythmias and those who are at risk of SCD (□ Antiarrhythmics, p.363).
- Diuretics—for patients with heart failure (□ Diuretics, p.380).

- Anticoagulation—for patients with AF and those at risk of thromboembolism (📖 Anticoagulants, p.375).
- The management of symptomatic patients with no obstruction can be very difficult.

Nonpharmacological treatments are aimed at ↓/relieving the obstruction in those with ASH who remain symptomatic despite pharmacological therapy. Treatment options might include the following:
- Alcohol-induced septal ablation (📖 Ablation, p.269)
- Dual-chamber pacing (📖 Types of pacing, p.224)
- Myectomy.

Further nonpharmacological management options might include the following:
- ICD insertion—for patients with symptomatic sustained ventricular arrhythmias or who are at high risk of SCD (📖 Implantable cardioverter-defibrillators, p.257)
- Cardiac transplantation
- Family screening—if familial disease is suspected.

Box 15.1 Criteria used to identify patients with HCM who are at highest risk of SCD
- Previous cardiac arrest
- Family history of premature SCD
- Hypotensive or flat BP response to exercise
- Unexplained syncope
- Non-sustained ventricular arrhythmia on Holter monitoring or on exercise
- Severe LVH of >30mm.

Dilated cardiomyopathy

Dilated cardiomyopathy (DCM) is essentially characterized by poorly con-
tracting and dilated ventricles, either the LV alone or both LV and RV
(Fig. 15.6), and affects 1 in 2500 of the population. DCM is generally more
common within the black population and is seen more frequently in ♂
than ♀.

Dilated ventricles with impaired systolic function are caused by factors
including hypertension, CHD, and valvular disease; however, in DCM, by
definition, all of these causes have been excluded and the disease is caused
by an intrinsic cardiac muscle problem.

In most cases, the cause is difficult to detect with certainty, in which
case the term 'idiopathic DCM' is used, there are, however, other factors
known to be associated with the development of DCM, these include:
- Familial/genetic disorders—including skeletal muscle disorders such as
  muscular dystrophies
- Myocardial inflammation, usually viral myocarditis
- Metabolic disorders (e.g. haemochromatosis and thyrotoxicosis)
- Autoimmune disease
- Pregnancy
- Infiltrative disorders
- Toxic substances (e.g. alcohol, chemotherapy, and recreational drugs)
- Nutritional deficiencies.

Clinical presentation

Patients generally present with symptoms of heart failure, such as fatigue,
dyspnoea, PND, orthopnoea, and peripheral oedema; other symptoms
include palpitations, syncope, and chest pain. Some patients might present with acute pulmonary oedema and, less commonly, an embolic event,
such as a systemic or pulmonary embolus, or sudden death. As with the
other cardiomyopathies, a patient could be diagnosed as a result of routine medical screening.

History
- Family history and pedigree
- Symptoms—chest pain, dizziness, SOB, palpitations
- Pregnancy.

Investigations

Similar to the other cardiomyopathies, investigations for DCM may
include the following:
- 12-lead ECG
- TTE (📖 Imaging studies: echocardiography, p.74)
- CXR (📖 Chest X-ray (CXR), p.64)
- Angiography (📖 Coronary angiography: preprocedure care, p.139)
- Advanced cardiac imaging (📖 Imaging studies: nuclear and cardiac
  magnetic resonance, p.76; Imaging studies: computed tomography
  calcium scoring, p.78)
- EPS (📖 Basic electrophysiology, p.263)
- Holter or ambulatory monitoring (📖 Ambulatory monitoring, p 72)
- ETT (📖 Exercise tolerance testing, p.71)

- Family screening and/or genetic testing if familial disease is suspected
- Cardiac biopsy (endomyocardial)
- Iron studies, CK, troponin, thyroid function.

Management

The 1° aim of treatment for patients with DCM is similar to that for all patients with heart failure, i.e. to control symptoms and prevent disease progression or complications, such as thromboembolism, progressive heart failure, and SCD.

Pharmacological management is outlined in Chapter 10 (📖 Clinical management, p.201), but can also include the following:
- Anticoagulation.

Non-pharmacological management could include the following options:
- Cardiac resynchronization therapy—to ensure the right and left ventricles contract simultaneously (📖 Clinical management, p.201)
- ICD insertion—for patients with EF <35% and symptomatic sustained ventricular arrhythmias (📖 Implantable cardioverter-defibrillators, p.257)
- Cardiac transplantation
- Family screening/genetic testing—if the disease could be familial.

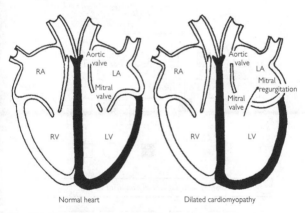

Fig. 15.6 Dilated cardiomyopathy. With kind permission from the Cardiomyopathy Association ℘ http://www.cardiomyopathy.org.

Arrhythmogenic right ventricular cardiomyopathy

ARVC is a genetically inherited disorder in which normal myocardial cells are replaced by fibro-fatty tissue. This may occur either in segments or affect the entire RV and/or part of the LV, and which progressively leads to heart failure. The estimated prevalence of ARVC is between 1 in 3000 and 1 in 10 000 of the population.

The pattern of inheritance of ARVC is either autosomal dominant or autosomal recessive. The most common pattern is autosomal dominant. As with HCM, a child has a 50:50 chance of inheriting the condition from an affected parent, thus only one abnormal gene is required to cause ARVC. However, in ARVC, having the mutated gene does not necessarily lead to the development of any features of the disease and thus an individual who does not develop the condition is an obligate carrier of the genetic mutation, which is referred to as 'incomplete penetrance' (Fig. 15.7).

In an autosomal-recessive pattern, an individual must inherit two copies of the genetic mutation, and thus both parents must be carriers. It is generally thought that the genetic mutations occur on the proteins desmoplakin and plakoglobin, which have important roles in linking myocardial cells together.

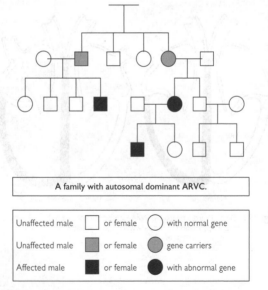

Fig. 15.7 Pedigree of autosomal dominant ARVC. With kind permission from the Cardiomyopathy Association ♫ http://www.cardiomyopathy.org.

History

• Family history (e.g. of sudden death) and pedigree
• Symptoms.

Clinical presentation

Patients might be asymptomatic or present with palpitations, presyncope, syncope, dyspnoea, including orthopnoea, and or peripheral oedema. Unfortunately, sudden death could also be the first manifestation of ARVC in some individuals. Similar to HCM, the severity of disease, symptoms, and risk of complications vary greatly between individuals with ARVC.

ARVC is often characterized by 'hot phases', in which the disease process is very apparent. The patient might experience sustained episodes of symptoms that include syncope and palpitations. During these phases, patients are at high risk of sudden death, but it is thought that between these phases the disease process is inactive.

Investigations

Investigations for ARVC can include the following:

• 12-lead ECG.
• Signal average ECG (SAECG)—multiple ECG tracings are obtained over ~20min. SAECG can detect high-frequency, low-amplitude electrical potentials that occur late in the QRS complex. These are known as late potentials. Presence of these identifies those at ↑ risk of ventricular arrhythmias.
• TTE (📖 Imaging studies: echocardiography, p.74).
• Holter or ambulatory monitoring (📖 Ambulatory monitoring, p.72).
• ETT (📖 Exercise tolerance testing, p.71).
• Angiography (📖 Coronary angiography: preprocedure care, p.139).
• EPS (📖 Basic electrophysiology, p.263).
• Endomyocardial biopsy.
• Implantable loop recorder.
• Advanced cardiac imaging (📖 Imaging studies: nuclear and cardiac magnetic resonance, p.76)
• Family screening and genetic testing.

Management

The general aims of management in patients with ARVC are to identify those who are at high risk of sudden death and offer protective measures, control symptoms, improve ventricular function, prevent or control cardiac arrhythmias, and screen family members.

Similar to HCM, an important part of the management of a patient with ARVC is risk stratification, with the intention of preventing sudden death.

Box 15.2 outlines the criteria which identifies those with ARVC who are at high risk of sudden death.

Management is tailored to an individual's symptoms and the risk of SCD. Treatment options can include the following:

- Antiarrhythmic drugs—for those with a cardiac arrhythmia (📖 Antiarrhythmics, p.363)
- ICD implantation—for those with life-threatening ventricular arrhythmias (📖 Implantable cardioverter-defibrillators, p.257)
- Heart failure therapies including anticoagulants (📖 Anticoagulants, p.375) in patients with severe right or biventricular systolic dysfunction
- Cardiac transplantation
- Family screening.

Box 15.2 Criteria used to identify patients with ARVC who are at high risk of sudden death
- Previous cardiac arrest
- History of syncope
- Evidence of ventricular arrhythmia on Holter monitoring or ETT
- A positive signal average ECG
- Family history of cardiac arrest
- Diffuse RV dilatation with a ↓ EF and evidence of LV involvement.

Restrictive cardiomyopathy

The least common of the cardiomyopathies, restrictive cardiomyopathy (RCM) is defined as a heart muscle disease that results in impaired ventricular filling with a normal or ↓ diastolic volume. The condition is usually a consequence of the myocardium becoming increasingly stiff, and resistance occurring in the filling phase of the cardiac cycle. Systolic function is generally normal, and the thickness of the ventricle walls may be normal or ↑, depending on the underlying cause. The condition can affect either or both ventricles and thus left and/or right heart failure may occur.

RCM may be idiopathic, familial, or 2° to systemic disorders, such as endomyocardial fibrosis, infiltrative disorders (e.g. amyloidosis and sarcoidosis), and metabolic disorders (e.g. Fabry's disease, carcinoid syndrome, Gaucher's disease, and mucopolysaccharidoses). RCM may also develop following radiotherapy for some types of cancer.

Clinical presentation

Patients with RCM generally present with symptoms of heart failure, such as dyspnoea, orthopnoea, PND, fatigue and weakness, peripheral oedema, ascites, cardiac conduction abnormalities (common in amyloidosis), palpitations, and thromboembolic complications.

Investigations

Investigations for RCM are similar to those of the other cardiomyopathies:
- 12-lead ECG
- TTE (📖 Imaging studies: echocardiography, p.74)
- Advanced cardiac imaging (📖 Imaging studies: nuclear and cardiac magnetic resonance, p.76; Imaging studies: computed tomography calcium scoring, p.78)
- Angiography (📖 Coronary angiography: preprocedure care, p.139)
- Endomyocardial biopsy
- Holter or ambulatory monitoring (📖 Ambulatory monitoring, p.72).

Management

The overall aims of management are to improve the symptoms of heart failure; treatments tend to be palliative and are similar to those for DCM and heart failure. Specific therapies might include the following:
- Medical therapies for heart failure (including possible anticoagulation)—(📖 Clinical management, p.201)
- Pacemaker insertion (📖 Permanent pacing management, p.236)—in patients with bradyarrhythmias 2° to AV conduction abnormalities
- Antiarrhythmic medications—for patients with rhythm disturbances (📖 Antiarrhythmics, p.363)
- Cardiac transplantation
- Family screening—if familial disease is suspected.

Nursing considerations

Nurses will probably encounter patients with cardiomyopathy at various stages in the disease process, and consequently, patients will require a variety of degrees of physical nursing care, advice, and support. Useful points for nurses to consider when managing any patient with cardiomyopathy are as follows:

- Monitor patients for complications of their cardiomyopathy (e.g. heart failure, rhythm disturbance, and thromboemboli) and report accordingly.
- Manage severe symptoms, such as heart failure, and sustained and symptomatic arrhythmias according to the evidence base.
- In patients with known ventricular arrhythmias, monitor K^+ levels, and aim to maintain at the level advised by the cardiology team.
- Be aware that some antiarrhythmic medications cardiomyopathy patients are commenced upon (e.g. amiodarone and sotalol) can prolong the QT interval, which might precipitate torsades de pointes (Polymorphic VT, p.251). Check the 12-lead ECG before commencing these drugs and before any ↑ in dose.
- Drug counselling—ensure that patients are aware of the actions and side effects of any medications, in particular advice regarding amiodarone (if applicable), which includes liver and thyroid function monitoring and ↑ photosensitivity (advise on the use of sun-blocking creams and avoiding bright sunlight to prevent skin damage).
- Nurses are often well placed to obtain family histories from patients so that a clear picture of any disease expression within the family can be identified.
- Nurses have a major role in offering advice and support to patients and their families. It is important to be aware that their diagnosis and subsequent lifestyle changes can have extensive social and emotional consequences, and can affect their relationships with other family members.
- Be prepared to deal with fear and anxiety—particularly in patients who are newly diagnosed.
- Information regarding their condition and treatment must be clear and timely. Provision of information and access to information can both help dispel misconceptions and enable patients to cope with their illness and can help those with cardiomyopathy adjust their lifestyle accordingly.
- Guide and advise patients on how to monitor for complications associated with their type of cardiomyopathy, and when to seek help whilst at home. In particular, patients should be aware of symptoms that could be life threatening, such as syncope and palpitations.
- Advise patients with ARVC of the potential for 'hot phases' and to seek urgent medical attention during these phases, so that appropriate treatment can be initiated.
- Patient should seek medical attention if they experience conditions that might lower K^+ levels or interfere with the absorption of medications (e.g. diarrhoea, vomiting, and poor appetite) and precipitate cardiac arrhythmias.

- Advise those who experience presyncope and syncope to avoid prolonged standing in hot conditions. Hot baths and showers should also be avoided because they can precipitate fainting.
- Provide advice on how patients can adapt their lifestyles—be aware that some patients with cardiomyopathy are discouraged from occupations in competitive sport, the police, commercial flying, vocational driving, and the military—any concerns must be discussed with their cardiologist.
- Provide general advice regarding diet—sensible eating is advised and weight loss is advised for those who are overweight, alcohol intake—moderation is advised because alcohol has a depressant effect on the heart. It is also advisable not to smoke.
- Patients with known rhythm disturbances should be cautioned against taking stimulants, including caffeine and recreational drugs, such as cocaine, ecstasy, and marijuana.
- Driving instructions—generally advice regarding driving should be sought from both the DVLA[1] and the cardiology team. Recommendations are generally made according to the patient's symptoms and stage of their cardiomyopathy.
- Provide advice regarding exercise. Recreational exercise is encouraged, however patients should be advised not to push themselves to their limit. If patients experience any palpitations, chest pain, or light-headedness when exercising, they should be advised to stop immediately. Be aware that some cardiomyopathy patients are advised not to take part in certain sports or strenuous activity because they are high risk of SCD and thus should seek medical advice regarding any exercise regimen.
- Be aware of the signs of anxiety and depression and discuss possible options for counselling and self-help groups; advise on relaxation techniques.
- Provide support and advice regarding family screening and genetic testing.
- Referral to appropriate specialist healthcare professionals if available.

---

[1] http://www.dvla.gov.uk

Related guidance

Cardiomyopathy Association—information booklets: ℘ http://www.cardiomyopathy.org

McMurray J, Adamopoulos S, Anker S, et al. (2012) ESC Guidelines for the diagnosis and treatment of acute and chronic heart failure 2012. European Heart Journal **33**, 1787–847.

National Institute for Health and Clinical Excellence (2010) *Chronic Heart Failure: Management of Chronic Heart Failure in Adults in Primary and Secondary Care*. Clinical Guideline 108. NICE, London.

National Institute for Health and Clinical Excellence (2011) *Chronic Heart Failure Quality Standards*. ℘ http://www.nice.org.uk/media/D6F/93/CHFQualityStandard.pdf

Other cardiac problems

Introduction

The most common problems that cardiac patients present with are related to CHD and valvular disorders. However, there are a number of infections and malignancies that can affect the heart and this chapter outlines the main disorders that can affect the pericardium and myocardium that are not covered elsewhere in the book.

There is also a brief section on heart disease in pregnancy.

Pericardial disease

The heart is enclosed in a sac called the pericardium which is made up of:
- A fibrous layer which is tough and inelastic ('fibrous pericardium').
- The serous pericardium which consists of two layers. The parietal layer lines the fibrous pericardium and the epicardium ('visceral layer') adheres to the outside of the heart.
- The pericardial space between the two layers normally contains ~15–30mL of serous fluid which ↓ friction as the heart beats.

The pericardium has several functions:
- It helps to anchor the heart inside the thorax and maintains its position.
- It is a barrier to infective organisms.
- It helps prevent the spread of malignancies from other organs.

Causes of pericardial disease include the following:
- Infection—viral, fungal, parasitic, or bacterial.
- Collagen and connective tissue diseases—e.g. systemic lupus erythematosus (SLE), polyarteritis nodosa, and scleroderma.
- Autoimmune disorders—rheumatoid arthritis, rheumatic fever, post-MI (Dressler's syndrome) and postcardiotomy syndromes.
- Acute MI.
- Bleeding into the pericardium—trauma, dissecting aortic aneurysm, or warfarin therapy.
- Neoplastic disease—usually invasive from other organs, e.g. lung, breast, or skin.
- Radiation.
- Hypothyroidism.
- Acute renal failure.
- Metabolic—uraemia or gout.
- Idiopathic—no known cause.

Pericardial disease has many causes but can be divided into three main types:
- Acute pericarditis (more common than chronic)
- Pericardial effusion
- Constrictive pericarditis.

Pericardial or cardiac tamponade is a medical emergency and is discussed in Chapter 18 (□ Cardiac tamponade, p.347).

Acute pericarditis

This is most commonly idiopathic, postsurgical, or a complication of MI. Pericarditis is also associated with underlying disease and could be the first presenting feature of diseases such as SLE.

Idiopathic pericarditis

Often occurs subsequent to an upper respiratory tract infection; generally, no causative organism is isolated, but a viral origin is presumed. Abrupt in onset and lasts 1–3wks.

Postcardiotomy syndromes

Usually seen 2–3wks after cardiac surgery, but can occur within a few days of the surgery. The syndrome usually lasts 2–4wks.

MI

Causes acute pericarditis in ~20% of patients. It commonly occurs 2–3 days post infarct, but can also occur as a late complication (weeks or months post infarct). The later presentation, known as Dressler's syndrome, is thought to be an autoimmune response and can recur.

Signs and symptoms

- Chest pain is the most common symptom. It is usually sudden in onset and described as 'sharp'. The pain around the chest is worse when the patient is lying or sitting back, with exacerbation on inspiration. It may be relieved when the patient sits forward.
- Tachypnoea is commonly associated with the pain, and patients often have a shallow breathing pattern.
- Pericardial friction rub is heard on auscultation—a grating noise is heard and remains when the patient holds their breath.
- Pyrexia—associated with the inflammatory process, although the patient's temperature does not usually exceed 39°C.
- Fatigue and malaise.
- Pericardial effusion.

Investigations

- 12-lead ECG—could show concave ST-segment elevation in all leads. After a few days, the T-wave inverts, but Q-waves are absent. ► Look for the different configuration of ST-segment elevation to differentiate acute MI, in which ST-segment elevation is convex.
- Echocardiogram—can detect pericardial effusion.
- Blood tests—ESR and white blood cell count are ↑. Troponin levels might be ↑ if pericarditis is associated with underlying myocarditis. C-reactive protein may also be ↑.
- CXR—↑ heart size, pulmonary oedema may be present.

Clinical management

- Pain management is the central therapeutic tool, with anti-inflammatory medication (e.g. ibuprofen or indomethacin) most commonly prescribed. If these are not effective colchicine may be used.

- Antitubercular medication is required for tuberculous pericarditis and the appropriate antibacterial agents are required if a causative organism is isolated.
- Antibiotics such as benzylpenicillin, flucloxacillin, or gentamicin are commonly prescribed if bacterial infection is suspected.
- Steroids may be considered.

Nursing considerations

The main principles of nursing care are as follows:
- Administer anti-inflammatory drugs and evaluate their effectiveness.
- Manage symptoms, such as pyrexia and pain.
- Monitor cardiovascular status.
- Support the patient's psychological needs. Pericarditis can commonly result from an underlying condition and the patient is likely to be anxious.

The following should be considered for patients with a diagnosis of acute pericarditis depending on the severity of symptoms:
- Record temperature at least every 4h—↑ frequency if patient feels feverish or if temperature ↑.
- Monitor BP and pulse to assess cardiovascular status at least every 4h—↑ frequency if symptoms deteriorate.
- Monitor respiratory rate and SaO₂ at least every 4h—administer supplemental O₂, as prescribed.
- Daily 12-lead ECG.
- Because the patient is relatively immobile during the acute phase, it is wise to measure and fit antiembolism stockings.
- Risk assessment for pressure ulcers is also indicated if the patient is immobile and feverish—implement preventive measures, depending on risk assessment score.

Pericardial effusion

This is the accumulation of fluid in the space between the layers of the pericardium. The fluid can have the following origin:
- Exudate of serous fluid or pus
- Transudate from heart failure
- Blood from trauma or malignant disease.

If the fluid builds up gradually, symptoms might be minimal because pericardial stretching can occur and cardiac function might not be compromised. Rapid accumulation of fluid can lead to cardiac tamponade (🕮 Cardiac tamponade, p.347) if the underlying cause is not identified and treated.

Signs and symptoms
- Pericardial-type pain might be present.
- Dyspnoea.
- Symptoms associated with an underlying condition—e.g. ascites and peripheral oedema in heart failure.

Investigations
- 12-lead ECG—shows ↓ voltage and tachycardia. Electrical alternans might be seen, whereby the complexes vary in amplitude from cycle to cycle. This reflects changes in the heart's position within the effusion and is highly suggestive of pericardial effusion.
- CXR—an enlarged cardiac silhouette is visible if >250mL of fluid has accumulated. An enlarged heart without evidence of pulmonary venous congestion makes the diagnosis of pericardial effusion probable.
- An echocardiogram can show excess fluid and the size of the effusion can be estimated. Serial Echos are helpful to observe progress of the effusion.

Clinical management
- No specific treatment is required for the effusion, but the underlying condition must be diagnosed and treated.
- Pericardiocentesis ('pericardial tap') might be required if the cause is not known because this can help to establish the nature of the effusion. Any fluid drawn should be sent for testing to rule out tuberculosis.

Nursing considerations
The main principles of nursing care are as follows:
- Manage symptoms of the underlying condition.
- Monitor cardiovascular status because cardiac tamponade is a possible *sequela* of pericardial effusion.
- Support the patient's psychological needs.

The following are considered for all patients who are diagnosed with pericardial effusion, but additional interventions relating to the underlying cause of the effusion might be required:

- Record temperature at least every 4h—↑ frequency if the patient feels feverish or if the temperature ↑.
- Monitor BP and pulse to assess cardiovascular status at least every 4h—↑ frequency if symptoms deteriorate.
- Monitor respiratory rate and SaO_2 at least every 4h—administer supplemental O_2, as prescribed.
- Daily 12-lead ECG.
- Monitor fluid status—either using a fluid-balance chart or by measuring the patient's weight daily.
- Observe neck veins for signs of ↑ JVP (📖 General assessment of the patient, p.27).

Constrictive pericarditis

This is usually caused by tuberculosis, mediastinal irradiation, previous surgery, or trauma. The pericardium becomes fibrosed and scarred, losing its elasticity. The heart becomes compressed, restricting cardiac filling. The presentation of constrictive pericarditis is similar to that of RVF.

Signs and symptoms
- ↓ CO and compensatory tachycardia
- Low pulse volume
- Engorged neck veins
- Hepatomegaly and ascites
- Peripheral oedema
- Pleuritic pain
- Dyspnoea.

Investigations
- 12-lead ECG—abnormal, but usually nonspecific, changes (e.g. low-voltage QRS). AF might be present.
- CXR—calcification might be seen. The heart is usually small or normal in size.
- Echocardiogram—pericardial thickening may be evident.
- CT or a CMR scan—can show pericardial thickening and reduces the need for a biopsy to differentiate between restrictive cardiomyopathy and constrictive pericarditis (☐ Imaging studies: nuclear and cardiac magnetic resonance, p.76; Imaging studies: computed tomography calcium scoring, p.78).
- Cardiac catheterization—abnormalities in diastolic chamber pressures are seen.
- Blood tests—usually show abnormal LFT and ↑ WBC count.

Clinical management
- Prevention is the best form of management. However, if severe pericardial constriction is evident, surgical pericardiectomy is required.

Nursing considerations
These relate mainly to the symptoms of right-sided failure that the patient presents with. The main principles of nursing care are as follows:
- Manage the symptoms of the condition.
- Monitor cardiovascular status.
- Support the patient's psychological needs, especially in relation to preparation for surgery.

The following are considered for all patients who are diagnosed with constrictive pericarditis, but additional interventions related to the underlying cause of the pericarditis (e.g. antitubercular therapy) and preparation for surgery are required (☐ Preoperative assessment, p.164):
- Monitor BP and pulse to assess cardiovascular status at least every 4h—↑ frequency if symptoms deteriorate.
- Monitor fluid status—either using a fluid-balance chart or by measuring the patient's weight daily.

- Observe neck veins for signs of ↑ JVP (□ General assessment of the patient, p.27).
- Risk assessment for pressure ulcers is also indicated if the patient is immobile—implement preventive measures, depending on risk assessment score.
- Antiembolism stockings are contraindicated if peripheral oedema is present.

Myocarditis

Myocarditis is inflammation of the myocardium. It causes a wide range of symptoms, from minor influenza-like symptoms to severe heart failure and sudden death. The causes of myocarditis are numerous (Box 16.1) and treatment greatly depends on the symptoms and aetiology. Often the cause is unknown and is attributed to a virus. There is a generalized inflammatory response, which can cause myocyte necrosis, and it is this part of the disease process that usually gives rise to clinical signs and symptoms. It is thought to have 3 phases:
- Phase 1—viral stage
- Phase 2—autoimmune phase
- Phase 3—DCM.

Box 16.1 Causes of myocarditis
- Viral (e.g. Rickettsia, Coxsackie B, mumps, hepatitis C and HIV)
- Fungal (e.g. candidiasis and aspergillosis)
- Bacterial (e.g. diphtheria, legionella, and salmonella)
- Protozoal (e.g. trypanosoma)
- Drug-induced (e.g. cocaine, arsenic, inotropes and reactions to drugs such as sulfonamides.)
- Others (e.g. radiation, peripartum, and autoimmunity)

Signs and symptoms

Variable and often nonspecific because of the aetiology, but patients seek medical help when the following occur:
- Chest pain
- Dyspnoea
- Palpitations
- Syncope
- Fatigue
- Fever

The most dramatic presentation will be acute DCM (🕮 Dilated cardiomyopathy, p.298).

Investigations

- 12-lead ECG—can reveal minor or major abnormalities.
- CXR—can show nonspecific abnormalities related to heart failure or cardiac enlargement.
- Echocardiogram—can identify cardiac dysfunction.
- Blood tests—↑ levels of cardiac markers are present because of myocyte damage. Viral titres can help to identify the causative organism.
- CMR imaging—helpful as a diagnostic tool for identifying myocarditis (🕮 Imaging studies: nuclear and cardiac magnetic resonance, p.76; Imaging studies: computed tomography calcium scoring, p.78).
- Biopsy—endomyocardial biopsy can help in the diagnosis, but it is costly and invasive.

Clinical management

- Restrict physical activity.
- Eradicate infective organism.
- Symptom management for arrhythmias and heart failure.
- In patients with severe haemodynamic compromise, an IABP, left ventricular assist device (LVAD) or ECMO might be required (Intra-aortic balloon pumps (IABPs), p.350; Ventricular assist devices, p.354; Extra corporeal membrane oxygenation, p.355.).

Nursing considerations

These relate mainly to the symptoms that the patient presents with. The main principles of nursing care are as follows:

- Manage the symptoms of the condition.
- Monitor cardiovascular status.
- Support the patient's psychological needs.

The following are considered for all patients who are diagnosed with myocarditis, but additional interventions related to the underlying cause (e.g. antibacterial therapy) are required.

- Initially continuous cardiac monitoring is advised to assess for signs of arrhythmias and ST changes.
- Monitor BP and pulse to assess cardiovascular status at least every 4h—↑ frequency if symptoms deteriorate.
- Record temperature at least every 4h.
- Monitor fluid status—either using a fluid-balance chart or by measuring the patient's weight daily to detect developing heart failure or evaluate treatment of heart failure.
- Observe neck veins for signs of ↑ JVP.
- Risk assessment for pressure ulcers is also indicated because the patient is immobile—implement preventive measures, depending on risk-assessment score.
- Antiembolism stockings are contraindicated if peripheral oedema is present.

Athlete's heart

The term 'athlete's heart' refers to normal physiological changes that occur as a result of prolonged cardiovascular exercise, which can simulate heart disease. The changes can include the following:

- ↑ left ventricular volume.
- ↓ resting HR.
- Slowing of AV nodal conduction, with first-degree AV nodal block seen on an ECG.
- LVH indicated on ECG.
- Incomplete RBBB on ECG.

If the athlete stops training, the heart returns to its previous condition. If changes as just outlined are noted, further investigations are warranted to rule out pathophysiological reasons for the changes.

Echocardiography is used to distinguish between athlete's heart and HCM. Because the person with athlete's heart does not have any symptoms, the signs are usually picked up when they are being treated for some unrelated medical or surgical condition. In these instances, the main nursing considerations are related to supporting the patient through any investigations and ensuring that they understand the reasons for these.

▶ Emphasise that the changes noted are physiological responses to prolonged exercise rather than pathophysiological changes that require treatment. Investigations are required to rule out any pathophysiological cause.

Preparticipation screening in young athletes

In some countries and some parts of the UK, preparticipation screening in young athletes is conducted to rule out conditions such as HCM, congenital defects, and arrhythmias, that may lead to SCD. While ECG changes may be due to athlete's heart, other areas such as episodes of syncope, chest pain, family history of cardiac disease, palpitations, ↑ BP, and excessive dyspnoea not related to exercise should all be investigated further.

Cardiac cancers

Cancer of the heart is extremely rare. However, nurses working in cardiac areas could care for patients with the following:

Myxoma

This is usually benign. Usually occurs in the LA and is a tumour attached to the septum by a pedicle. Thus, its position can vary with posture and so associated symptoms might be transient. Symptoms are usually related to obstruction of the MV and resemble those of MS (Mitral valve stenosis, p.88). Diagnosis is made from an echocardiogram and surgical intervention is required.

Carcinoid syndrome

Malignant carcinoid tumours, with liver metastases, can be associated with stenosis and regurgitation of the pulmonary and tricuspid valves. The mechanism of the valve lesion is not fully understood, but it is thought to be related to secretion of kinins by the tumour. However, symptoms of right-sided heart failure can be present and these are treated using conventional therapy (Clinical management, p.201).

Carcinoma-related pericardial effusions

Pericardial effusion can result from fluid infiltration from adjacent lung or breast tumours in patients with advanced-stage disease. Treatment is palliative and related to symptom management.

Heart disease in pregnancy

Heart disease is the leading cause of maternal death in the UK. Some of the reasons for this include CAD, ↑ maternal age, obesity, and type 2 diabetes. More women with congenital heart disease are also surviving to adulthood and although pregnancy can be tolerated well with many congenital heart defects, there are some that pose higher risks to both the mother and the fetus.

Normal haemodynamic changes during pregnancy include the following:
- ↑ CO (due to an ↑ SV and HR)
- ↓ SVR
- ↑ ventricular chamber mass
- Pro-arrhythmic state due to ↑ catecholamines and hormonal changes
- ↑ Hypercoagulability.

The most dramatic haemodynamic changes occur during labour, delivery, and the early postpartum period.

The ESC has produced guidelines on the management of CVD in pregnancy. Some of the essential messages are as follows:[1]

General

- Counselling of women with known or suspected CVD should start before pregnancy and include genetic counselling.
- High-risk women should be managed in specialist centres.
- Suspected fetal congenital malformations in affected families should have an Echo from week 13.
- Diagnostic tests involving radiation should be avoided (Echo, exercise test, or MRI [without contrast] preferred).
- Cardiac catheter and surgery avoided in pregnancy where possible.
- Vaginal delivery preferred.

Congenital heart disease

- Risk of pregnancy depends on disease, ventricular and valve function, and cyanosis.
- Individualized plan of follow-up should be devised.
- Pregnancy is usually contraindicated in pulmonary ↑ BP or Eisenmenger syndrome (Ⅲ Eisenmenger syndrome, p.285).

Aortic diseases

- Pregnancy can be high risk for those with an aortic pathology.
- Dissection mostly occurs in last trimester or early postpartum.
- Pregnancy discouraged in Marfan's syndrome or when aortic root is >45mm.
- Caesarean advised if aortic diameter is >45mm.

Valve disease

- Moderate and severe MS should be treated pre pregnancy as poorly tolerated.
- Regurgitant lesions better tolerated than stenotic.
- For those with mechanical valves oral anticoagulant with vitamin K antagonist are safest.

Coronary artery disease

- PPCI (with bare metal stent) is the treatment of choice in ACS/STEMI.
- Pregnancy is usually ok in known CHD if no residual ischaemia and LVEF >40%.

Cardiomyopathy

- Pregnancy is usually tolerated well in HCM.
- There is a risk of deterioration in DCM.
- Peripartum cardiomyopathy is usually suspected if there is LV systolic dysfunction without identifiable cause in the last month of pregnancy or first months postpartum.

Arrhythmias

- May become more frequent during pregnancy or may manifest for the first time.
- If the mother is haemodynamically unstable with an arrhythmia cardioversion should be considered.
- AVNRT or AVRT—vagal manoeuvres or adenosine should be considered.

Hypertension

- Drug treatment of severe ↑ BP is beneficial.
- Methyldopa is the recommended drug of choice in the long-term management of ↑ BP in pregnancy.
- ACE inhibitors, angiotensin II antagonists, and direct renin inhibitors are contraindicated in pregnancy.

[1] European Society of Cardiology (2011) *Essential Messages from ESC Guidelines: Cardiovascular Diseases During Pregnancy.* http://www.escardio.org/guidelines-surveys/esc-guidelines/Pages/cardiovascular-diseases-during-pregnancy.aspx

Related guidance

Cooper LT, Baughman KL, Feldman AM, et al. (2007) The role of endomyocardial biopsy in the management of cardiovascular disease. A scientific statement from the American Heart association, American College of Cardiology and the European Society of Cardiology. *European Heart Journal* **28**, 3076–93.

Regitz-Zagrosek V, Blomstrom Lundqvist C, Borghi C, et al. (2011) ESC guidelines on the management of cardiovascular diseases during pregnancy. *European Heart Journal* **32**, 3147–97.

Cardiac rehabilitation

Introduction

The risk factors for CVD and their suggested management are discussed in Chapter 1 (◻ Nonmodifiable risk factors, p.11; Modifiable risk factors: 1, p.12) along with the role of health promotion (◻ Behaviour change, p.19). This chapter looks at the role of cardiac rehabilitation for those at risk of cardiac disease or who have sustained a cardiac event.

Cardiac rehabilitation was one of the few areas of the National Service Framework for Coronary Heart Disease where targets were not all met. It is now one of the priority areas for NHS Improvement Heart.

Cardiac rehabilitation

All patients who have had a cardiac event should be offered cardiac rehabilitation. This can start before admission, for those patients that are being admitted for cardiac surgery or an intervention, at a pre-admission clinic, or while the patient is on the waiting list. However, it usually commences during the in-patient stay. Cardiac rehabilitation was previously divided into four phases but recently a different pathway for cardiac rehabilitation has been proposed[1] (see Fig. 17.1). Whereas most Trusts might employ cardiac rehabilitation nurses, it is the responsibility of all nurses to participate in the rehabilitation process when the opportunity presents itself.

Standards and core components of cardiac rehabilitation

The British Association for Cardiovascular Prevention and Rehabilitation has produced standards and core components for disease prevention and rehabilitation (Box 17.1).[2]

The core components are:
- Health behaviour change and education
- Lifestyle risk factor management—physical activity and exercise, diet, smoking cessation
- Psychosocial health
- Medical risk factor management
- Cardioprotective therapies
- Long-term management
- Audit and evaluation.

Patients should be identified and referred to the cardiac rehabilitation team as soon as possible. Regardless of whether the patient is willing or able to participate in a formal exercise programme they will still need information and reassurance about their condition. It is important to remember that immediately after a cardiac event the patient might not be in a position to take in too much information, so all verbal information should be supported by appropriate written literature. The family should be included where possible. Referral to other services (e.g. dietician, smoking cessation advisor, psychologist) might be required following assessment of cardiac rehabilitation needs.

Box 17.1 Standards for cardiac rehabilitation

1. The delivery of the seven core components employing an evidence-based approach
2. An integrated multidisciplinary team consisting of qualified and competent practitioners, led by a clinical coordinator
3. Identification, referral, and recruitment of eligible patient populations
4. Early initial assessment of individual patient needs in each of the core components, ongoing assessment, and re-assessment upon programme completion
5. Early provision of a cardiac rehabilitation programme, with a defined pathway of care which meets the core components and is aligned with patient preference and choice
6. Registration and submission of data to the National Audit for Cardiac Rehabilitation (NACR)
7. Establishment of a business case including a cardiac rehabilitation budget which meets the full service costs.

Reproduced from British Association for Cardiovascular Prevention and Rehabilitation Standards and Core Components for Cardiovascular Disease Prevention and Rehabilitation 2012 (2nd edn).

[1] Department of Health (2010) *Service Specification for Cardiac Rehabilitation Services*. Department of Health, London.

[2] British Association for Cardiovascular Prevention and Rehabilitation (2012) *The BACPR Standards and Core Components for Cardiovascular Disease Prevention and Rehabilitation 2012* (2nd edition). British Cardiovascular Society, London.

Delivery of cardiac rehabilitation

Traditionally patients were invited to an out-patient cardiac rehabilitation programme 4–6 weeks after a cardiac event such as ACS or CABG. However, the recommendation is that patients should now be engaged in relevant aspects of cardiac rehabilitation within 2–3 weeks of diagnosis or discharge from hospital. During this period patients are likely to be receptive to advice regarding lifestyle changes. Depression, anxiety, and social isolation can also be issues, which cardiac rehabilitation can help to address. An assessment of the patient should normally take place to assess their suitability for exercise, patient goals with regard to cardiac rehabilitation, and to plan an appropriate programme of care (Fig. 17.1).

Rehabilitation should be menu based and designed to meet the needs of the individual patient. It may include the following aspects:

- Telephone support, in the form of follow-up calls or helpline services
- Home visits by a specialist cardiac nurse
- Drop-in or organized outpatient clinics
- Web-based programmes
- Literature
- Community-based or hospital-based exercise programmes
- Home-based programmes such as the Heart Manual[3] or Angina Plan[4] with monitoring and support from cardiac rehabilitation staff
- Some programmes may be run by community centres, charities, private organizations, and sport centres, particularly for long-term exercise maintenance.

Traditionally, cardiac rehabilitation programmes were only offered to patients following either MI or CABG. Although centres should now be offering rehabilitation to all eligible cardiac patients, it is suggested that high priority should be given to those following ACS, post reperfusion, chronic heart failure, or those with device insertion for ACS or heart failure.

Evidence suggests that the more encouragement patients are given to attend an exercise programme, the more likely they are to participate. Even if patients are not able to exercise, it is important that they are given appropriate advice regarding their individual risk factors. This advice needs to be practical, realistic, and achievable. There are a number of resources available to help health professionals develop and deliver cardiac rehabilitation (see 📖 Related guidance, p.332).

Re-assessment of the patient should take place at the end of a structured exercise programme followed by a long-term management plan.

Long-term follow-up

Some patients may carry on to attend a community-based cardiac rehabilitation programme. There are also a number of patient-led support groups that can be beneficial. Long-term follow-up may include auditing of risk factors, such as smoking cessation rates, in addition to morbidity and mortality figures. This auditing may be carried out by the patient's GP practice.

Auditing of cardiac rehabilitation

Each cardiac rehabilitation programme is expected to audit and evaluate their service. In England, Wales, and Northern Ireland this information is collected by the National Audit of Cardiac Rehabilitation and an annual report is produced.

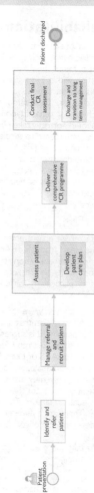

Sharing cardiac rehabilitation information (education) and long-term management strategy with the patient

*CR = cardiac rehabilitation

Fig. 17.1 Pathway for cardiac rehabilitation. Department of Health (2010) *Service Specification for Cardiac Rehabilitation Services*. Department of Health, London. Used with permission under the Open Government Licence.

3 NHS Lothian (2012) *The Heart Manual*. ℘ http://www.theheartmanual.com (accessed 25 October 2012).

4 ℘ http://www.anginaplan.org.uk (accessed 25 October 2012).

Management of lifestyle and risk factors

The goals of lifestyle management are as follows:
- Improve quality of life.
- Help to control symptoms, such as SOB, lethargy, and chest pain.
- Reduce the risk of a further cardiac event or death.
- ↑ the lifespan of CABG/PCI

To achieve these goals, many patients might need help with changing behavioural risk factors (📖 Behaviour change, p.19). It is important that patients are motivated to change behaviour that has a negative effect on their health and that they set realistic goals to achieve this. If the patient has a number of risk factors, such as the need to stop smoking and lose weight, advice regarding priorities might be required.

Nurses can help patients to set goals/objectives for behavioural change. However, it is vital that these are the patient's goals and not those of the healthcare professional. The role of the nurse is to provide the patient with relevant information and encouragement to achieve their goals. It is important that the goals set are realistic, achievable, and measurable. For example, if weight loss is the target, the patient needs to decide how much weight they want to lose and the period of time in which they will achieve the weight loss. They also need to think about how they will achieve this (e.g. by committing to an exercise programme, joining a slimming club, etc.). The nurse can help with setting goals and providing advice on sensible weight loss. To ↑ motivation, it is important that the patient includes a system of rewards for achieving their goals. The aim should be for lifestyle changes to become permanent and the emphasis should be on finding practical and enjoyable solutions so that the patient does not feel deprived.

Often, small changes in behaviour will result in a positive effect on a person's health. Although the patient might only be focusing on one area, such as weight loss, this can also lead to an improvement in physical fitness, ↓ BP, and ↓ blood cholesterol levels.

Advice on reducing risk factors for CVD can be found in Chapter 1.

Physical activity

Physical activity can help to ↓ BP, ↑ HDL cholesterol, ↓ a person's risk of a stroke, help prevent or control diabetes, aid weight loss, and improve the chances of survival following a heart attack. It also has a positive effect on depression, anxiety, and improves well-being. It is therefore an important part of rehabilitation and 2° prevention. Physical activity should be part of daily activities and whilst some individuals may find it beneficial to join a gym or a formal exercise class, this is not necessary or appropriate for all. Following a cardiac event, individuals should seek medical advice prior to undertaking any strenuous exercise.

Physical activity levels will depend on the symptoms the patient is experiencing and any other comorbidities, such as arthritis or respiratory conditions that may limit activity. However, individual programmes can be tailored to suit the patient's needs. An ETT may be used as a guide to the level of exercise that is safe for an individual to do.

Walking is an activity that most patients will be able to do and if done regularly will help improve fitness levels. Other aerobic activities include cycling, swimming, and dancing. General advice for those who are ↑ their physical activity includes the following:

- Activities should include a warm-up and cool-down period.
- Those patients who experience angina should carry GTN spray or tablets with them (in some cases it may be advisable for individuals to take GTN prior to any exercise).
- Activity should be stopped if the individual experiences chest pain, dizziness, acute SOB, or palpitations.
- Activity levels should be ↑ gradually. The time spent doing the activity, the intensity, and the distance (or duration) can be ↑ if the individual has not experienced any problems with the activity.
- Those with angina should not exercise in very cold weather or immediately after a heavy meal.
- It is better for the individual to try and do small amounts frequently. The aim is to build up to 30min of moderately intense activity in a day on at least 5 days of the week. The 30min can be broken into shorter sessions, e.g. three sessions each of 10min.
- The 'talk test' can be used as a way for individuals to check if they are exercising at the right intensity. The aim is that the individual should still be able to talk but will feel warm and be breathing heavily. If they cannot talk whilst exercising they are working too hard and should slow down.

Sex

Patients might be anxious about resuming sexual activity following a cardiac event. However, it is suggested that if an individual can climb a flight of stairs they should be able to participate in sexual activity. Some medications (e.g. β-blockers) can affect sexual performance (🕮 β blockers, p.366). Patients should discuss their concerns with their GP or cardiologist.

Return to work

Returning to work following a cardiac event may be influenced by the following factors:

- Age
- Other comorbidities
- Economic status
- Attitude of patient and family
- Type of work (e.g. heavy manual labour would not be advisable post MI or post cardiac surgery)
- Attitude of physician
- Attitude of employer
- Recurrence of symptoms.

Psychosocial assessment

Patients may experience depression, anxiety, and social isolation after a cardiac event. Although this is quite normal, and is usually temporary, in some patients it can be more severe and can have a negative effect on their recovery. A basic psychosocial assessment should be performed on all patients while they are in hospital, and if necessary, the patient should be referred to a psychologist. There are a variety of tools (often questionnaires) that can be used to explore the patient's psychological and emotional needs and quality of life.

Related guidance

American Heart Association (2011) Referral, enrolment and delivery of cardiac rehabilitation/secondary prevention programmes at clinical centers and beyond. *Circulation* **124**, 2951–60.

British Association for Cardiovascular Prevention and Rehabilitation (2012) *The BACPR Standards and Core Components for Cardiovascular Disease Prevention and Rehabilitation 2012* (2nd edition). British Cardiovascular Society, London.

British Heart Foundation (2010) *What Should I Expect from Cardiac Rehabilitation – A Guide for Heart Patients in England*. BHF, London.

Department of Health (2010) *Coronary Heart Disease and the Need for Cardiac Rehabilitation*. Department of Health, London.

Department of Health (2010) *Planning a Cardiac Rehabilitation Service*. Department of Health, London.

Department of Health (2010) *Service Specification for Cardiac Rehabilitation Services*. Department of Health, London.

National Audit of Cardiac Rehabilitation (2012) *Annual Statistics Report 2011*. BHF, York.

NHS Improvement Heart (2010) *Transforming Cardiac Rehabilitation: Celebrating Achievements and Sharing the Learning from the National Projects*. NHS Improvement, London.

National Institute for Health and Clinical Excellence (2011) *Cardiac Rehabilitation Services (Commissioning Guide)*. NICE, London.

Perk J, DeBacker G, Gohlke H, *et al.* (2012) European guidelines on cardiovascular disease prevention in clinical practice. *European Heart Journal* **33**, 1635–701.

Taylor R, Dalal H, Jolly K, Moxham T, Zawada A (2010) Comparisons of different modes of cardiac rehabilitation. Cochrane Database of Systematic Reviews **1**, CD007130. doi: 10.1002/14651858. CD007130.pub2.

Chapter 18

Cardiovascular emergencies

Introduction

Cardiovascular emergencies are either sudden events or are preceded by a noticeable deterioration in the patient's condition. Although critically ill patients are usually cared for in a specialist unit (e.g. CCU, HDU, ITU) it is becoming more common for these patients to be found on general wards. Many hospitals will have outreach teams to facilitate the appropriate care of these patients and provide support for the staff looking after them. Patients who develop symptoms of ACS on a non-cardiac ward are not always assessed and managed appropriately, which can put them at high risk. This chapter discusses the assessment of the deteriorating patient, resuscitation, and the causes and treatment of some cardiovascular emergencies.

Assessment of the deteriorating patient

Many in-hospital cardiac arrests could potentially be prevented if it is noted that a patient's condition is deteriorating and that appropriate interventions are then put in place. Changes in observations, in particular respiratory rate, can be an early indication of deterioration; however, this is not always recorded accurately or frequently. Use an ABCDE approach to assess the patient:

- Airway
- Breathing
- Circulation
- Disability
- Exposure.

Many trusts use a scoring system, such as a medical early warning system, to highlight patients who are at risk of deterioration and who may need assessment or intervention by a critical care outreach team.

Airway

An assessment of the airway includes detection of signs of partial or full airway obstruction. This may include the following:

- No sound—this could indicate full obstruction
- Snoring
- Gurgling
- Gasping
- Obvious visual obstruction
- Oedema
- Swelling
- Bleeding.

Simple airway manoeuvres, such as head tilt/chin lift, may open the airway and relieve the obstruction. If a neck injury is suspected, use a jaw thrust to prevent damage to the cervical spine. Suction might be required for fluids, such as blood, vomit, or excess saliva. Only remove dentures if they are loose or ill-fitting and likely to cause an obstruction. An airway adjunct, such as a nasal or oropharyngeal airway, can also be used to support the airway. Do not use nasal airways if a skull fracture is suspected (e.g. bruising around ears and eyes or cerebrospinal fluid leaking from the nose or ears). Only use oropharyngeal airways if the person is deeply unconscious.

Breathing

A full description of respiratory assessment is found in (🕮 Respiratory assessment, p.57). In a deteriorating patient, assess the following:

- Rate, rhythm, and depth of respirations (<10 breaths/min or >30 breaths/min indicates a problem).
- Use of accessory muscles to help breathing.
- Breath sounds—listen for gurgling, wheezes, and crackles.
- Equal air entry—causes of unequal air entry include pneumothorax, consolidation, and basal collapse.

- Chest symmetry.
- Position of the trachea.
- Evidence of peripheral or central cyanosis.
- Complaints of SOB or difficulty breathing.
- O_2 saturation levels.

If O_2 is required it should be given (>10L/min) through a mask with a reservoir bag attached to maintain SaO_2 as close to normal as possible.

Circulation

In addition to cardiovascular observations, the assessment of circulation includes looking for any obvious signs of bleeding. The following should be included:

- HR, rhythm, and volume.
- BP.
- 12-lead ECG.
- Observation of neck veins to see if they are full or collapsed and CVP, if available.
- Urine output (should be >0.5mL/kg of body weight/h) and fluid balance.
- Evidence of bruising, swelling, redness, bleeding, or pain.
- Observation of wound sites, if present.
- Capillary refill—assess by applying pressure to the fingertip for 5s. When the pressure is released, the skin should resume normal colour within 2s.
- Colour and temperature of the skin.
- Palpate central and peripheral pulses (unable to palpate peripheral pulses if systolic BP <80mmHg).

Disability

Neurological status is assessed initially using the alert, responsive to voice, responsive to pain, or unresponsive scale (AVPU). A more in-depth assessment, such as the Glasgow Coma Scale, can follow. The FAST can be used to assess for stroke (facial weakness, arm weakness, and speech problems).[1] Also, assess blood sugar and consider any other factors that could affect level of consciousness, such as hypoxia, poor perfusion, and the effects of any drugs taken.

Exposure

At this point, consider any other factors not previously considered that could cause the patient's condition to deteriorate. If not already recorded, take the patient's temperature. Check the body for signs such as bruising, haematomas, track marks from needles, etc.

---

[1] The Stroke Association website. ℘ http://www.stroke.org.uk (accessed 25 October 2012).

Basic life support

Out of hospital

An algorithm for adult basic life support out of hospital is shown in Fig. 18.1.

In hospital

An algorithm for adult in-hospital resuscitation is shown in Fig. 18.2.

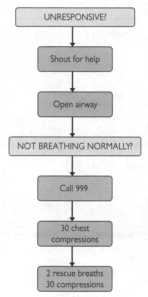

Fig. 18.1 Adult basic life-support algorithm (2010). Reproduced with kind permission of the Resuscitation Council (UK).

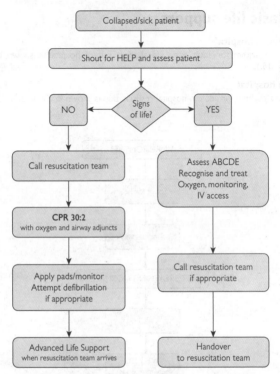

Fig. 18.2 In-hospital resuscitation (2010). Reproduced with kind permission of the Resuscitation Council (UK).

Resuscitation

The current guidelines for in-hospital resuscitation are outlined earlier in this chapter (Fig. 18.2). In the event of a cardiac arrest the following are vital:

• Recognize collapsed patients.
• Initiate basic life support as soon as possible, in particular chest compressions.
• Call for further help.
• Defibrillation (where indicated) should be done ASAP (within 3min).

A number of people can usually assist, but a coordinated approach is important to ensure that resuscitation is started quickly.

The initial assessment of the patient involves establishing their level of consciousness and then opening the airway, looking for signs of airway obstruction, and assessing signs of breathing and circulation. Assessment of breathing and circulation can be performed at the same time but should not take more than 10s. If it is established that the patient is not breathing and does not have a pulse, then one person should go and call the cardiac arrest team and then bring the resuscitation trolley to the bedside, while another performs CPR. 30 compressions should be followed by 2 ventilations. Perform compressions at a rate of at least 100 compressions/min (not more than 120) and a depth of 5cm. Ventilations should be performed using a pocket mask or a bag–mask–valve system (whichever is closer to hand). The bag–mask–valve system might require two people: one person to hold the mask in place and ensure a tight seal, and the second person to squeeze the bag. Change the person performing the compressions frequently because they can be very tiring.

Check the contents of the trolley at least once daily, replacing items as necessary and keeping them in working order. All nurses must familiarize themselves with the procedure for calling the cardiac arrest team.

Start cardiac monitoring, by either monitoring electrodes or defibrillation pads, as soon as possible so that the underlying cardiac arrest rhythm can be established.

Cardiac arrest rhythms include asystole (Fig. 18.3), ventricular fibrillation (VF, Fig. 18.4), ventricular tachycardia (VT, Fig. 18.5), or pulseless electrical activity (PEA).

VF is a chaotic uncoordinated rhythm (📖 Ventricular fibrillation, p.253) that might respond to defibrillation. Pulseless VT (📖 Ventricular tachycardia, p.251) should also be defibrillated. Asystole means that there is no electrical activity. If asystole is suspected, check the leads to ensure they are connected and also check the gain on the monitor to ensure that it is not fine VF. Defibrillation is not indicated for asystole. Asystole has the worst prognosis in terms of resuscitation. Reversible causes should be investigated (📖 Reversible causes, p.341). PEA exists if a rhythm normally associated with a cardiac output is seen on the monitor but the patient does not have a pulse. It is often caused when the electrical activity of the heart is working but physically the heart cannot pump, e.g. in the presence of cardiac tamponade (📖 Cardiac tamponade, p.347) or tension pneumothorax (📖 Tension pneumothorax, p.346). Treatment of the rhythm includes CPR and correcting the underlying cause. Defibrillation is not suggested.

When the resuscitation team arrives it is important that information is given to them in a structured way. Many centres use either SBAR (Situation, Background, Assessment, Recommendation) or RSVP (Reason, Story, Vital Signs, Plan).[2]

▶ Attend to the needs of other patients during a cardiac arrest because this is a distressing experience for them. If relatives are present, they might wish to stay with the patient during the resuscitation. This should be handled sensitively and a nurse should stay with them. If the patient's next of kin is not present, contact them as soon as possible.

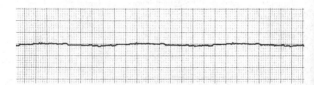

Fig. 18.3 Asystole.

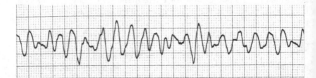

Fig. 18.4 Ventricular fibrillation.

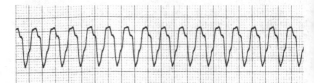

Fig. 18.5 Ventricular tachycardia.

[2] ℘ http://www.resus.org.uk

Advanced life support

Advanced life support (ALS) includes advanced airway management, defibrillation (if indicated), drug administration, and identifying and treating reversible causes. Fig. 18.6 shows the algorithm for ALS in the UK.

Drug administration

The most common drugs used in resuscitation are adrenaline and amiodarone (for VF and periarrest rhythms). Adrenaline (1mg) is administered IV once chest compressions have re-started after the 3rd shock and then every 3–5min to improve perfusion to the brain and heart. IV access must be established as soon as possible and IV fluids can also be given (with caution in some patients).

Advanced airway management

When the anaesthetist (or other appropriately competent person) arrives, the patient is usually intubated to secure the airway and improve oxygenation. This may be with an endotracheal tube or laryngeal mask airway.

Reversible causes

A number of reversible causes might have led to the cardiac arrest (see Fig. 18.6). Some of these causes are discussed in more detail in this chapter. Blood tests are required to check for electrolyte levels and the presence of toxins.

National Cardiac Arrest Audit (NCAA)

NCAA is a UK wide database of in-hospital cardiac arrests. It is important that audit data of each cardiac arrest is collected to help in the prevention and management of future cardiac arrests.

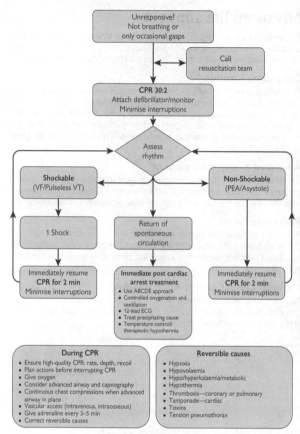

Fig. 18.6 Adult advanced life support algorithm (2012). Reproduced with kind permission of the Resuscitation Council (UK).

Defibrillation

Defibrillation can improve outcomes from VT/VF, ∴ early defibrillation is vital and there is ↑ emphasis in the latest resuscitation guidelines on the importance of not delaying the first shock.[3] Defibrillation can either be performed using a manual defibrillator or an automated external defibrillator (AED). Defibrillation aims to stop arrhythmias and enable the SA node to take over the rhythm again. Defibrillation is extremely dangerous if individuals are in contact with the patient or the patient's bed during the shock. The operator must ensure that everyone stands clear before shocking the patient and if O_2 is delivered via a face mask this should be moved away to minimize the risk of sparks causing a fire (less risk with adhesive pads than with paddles).

AEDs

AEDs enable defibrillation to take place without the operator needing to interpret the rhythm. Pads are placed on the patient which allow for the ECG to be analysed by the AED. ▶ It is important that contact with the skin is enhanced so it must be dry, and in some cases hair may need to be shaved. If a shockable rhythm is found, the machine charges up and advises the user to shock (semi-automatic AED) or delivers the shock (automatic AED). This can only take place after the operator has established it is safe to do so.

AEDs have been placed in public places, such as shopping centres, airports, and stations, to enable fast access to defibrillation. They are also widely used in hospitals so it is important that as many nurses as possible are trained to use them.

Manual defibrillation

Manual defibrillation requires the user to have an understanding of rhythm abnormalities. The operator must ensure that the area is clear before charging the defibrillator and shocking the patient. Defibrillators can be monophasic or biphasic. If they are monophasic, the energy selected for the shock should be 360J. Biphasic defibrillators vary (refer to manufacturer's guidelines) but should usually be set at 150–200J, with subsequent shocks at 150–360J.

Many machines now have pads instead of paddles. ▶ However, if paddles are in use, apply gel pads first.

---

3 ℘ http://www.resus.org.uk

Pulmonary embolism

PE and DVT are two clinical presentations of venous thromboembolism (VTE). DVT in the leg causes ~90% of all PE. It can also be caused by fat embolism, tumour, air embolism, or foreign matter. PEs are often missed or incorrectly diagnosed because the symptoms are similar to other problems, such as MI. The risk factors for VTE include the following:

- ↑ age
- Previous VTE
- Major surgery (in particular abdominal surgery or hip or knee replacement)
- Pregnancy
- Chronic heart or respiratory failure
- Lower limb fracture
- Prolonged hospitalization

Signs and symptoms

The signs and symptoms exhibited depend on the size of the embolus. A PE can be acute or chronic depending on the onset of symptoms. If only a small embolus is present, the patient might complain of lethargy and mild SOB. A medium embolus (occlusion of a segment of the pulmonary artery tree) can lead to haemoptysis, chest pain, pyrexia, and SOB. A massive PE (occlusion of >2/3 of the pulmonary artery bed) leads to signs of right heart failure, ↓ CO, ↑ CVP, signs of cyanosis, and ↑ HR. The patient might collapse and present with cardiac arrest.

Investigations

NICE guidance[4] suggests that if a PE is suspected treatment should be given within 4h and investigative tests should be carried out within 24h. Investigations are carried out depending on the clinical probability of PE. There are scoring systems available such as the Wells score that can be used to determine the likelihood of PE.[4] Some investigations are not useful when there is a high probability of PE as this would not change the management.

- CXR—to rule out other causes of acute SOB, such as pneumothorax.
- ECG—the main finding is sinus tachycardia. This could also show S1Q3T3 pattern (a deep S-wave in lead I, Q wave in lead III, and an inverted T-wave in lead III). It is not always present and absence should not rule out PE. This pattern is often associated with a massive PE. There could also be RBBB, atrial arrhythmias, RAH, right axis deviation, and non-specific ST and T changes anteriorly.
- ABG.
- Blood tests to include FBC, U&E and D-dimer assay. D-dimer assay is not useful in those with high probability of PE however a −ve D-dimer can rule out PE in patients with a low or intermediate clinical probability of PE.
- CT pulmonary angiography.
- Ventilation—perfusion (VQ) scan.
- Echo—particularly for those with high clinical probability of PE.
- Lower limb ultrasound

Recent guidance[4] suggests that investigations for cancer should be carried out in people <40yrs who develop a PE with no clear cause. (Those with cancer have 4-fold risk of thromboembolism.) Tests should include serum calcium, LFTs, abdo-pelvic CT scan, and mammography for women.

Treatment

Management depends on the size of the embolus and the clinical condition of the patient. If the patient presents in right heart failure or cardiogenic shock treat accordingly (□ Left-sided or right-sided heart failure, p.196, Cardiogenic shock, p.349). Treatment options for a large PE with a high risk of mortality include thrombolysis or pulmonary embolectomy. Other management options include fondaparinux, SC LMWH, unfractionated heparin, oral anticoagulation (to maintain an INR of 2–3) or thrombolytics. Anticoagulation may be continued for approximately 2–3mths, unless the DVT/PE is recurrent, in which case anticoagulant treatment is lifelong.

Prevention of VTE

More emphasis has been placed on the prevention of VTE in recent years. Nurses should ensure that all patients admitted to hospital have been risk assessed for the potential of VTE developing and appropriate measures put in place, e.g. pharmacological prophylaxis, antiembolism stockings. Guidelines have been produced by NICE, SIGN, and ESC (see □ Related guidance, p.359).

[4] National Institute for Health and Clinical Excellence (2012) *Venous Thromboembolic Diseases: the Management of Venous Thromboembolic Diseases and the Role of Thrombophilia Testing*. NICE, London.

Tension pneumothorax

Tension pneumothorax occurs when air enters the pleural space but has no way of escaping. Tension builds up in the area, which leads to a shift within the mediastinum. This can eventually cause pressure on the heart, which might stop beating. This is often one of the reasons for PEA in cardiac arrest. If blood is present in the pleural space, this is a haemothorax.

Causes

Pneumothorax sometimes occurs spontaneously, particularly in young ♂. It can occur following chest drain removal or because of cardiac trauma, such as a road traffic accident or fighting. It can also occur because of artificial ventilation, particularly in those who have high airway pressures.

Signs and symptoms

- Acute SOB.
- ↓ or no air entry on the affected side.
- Tachycardia.
- The patient might become distressed.
- There might be obvious signs of injury to the chest.
- Hyper-resonance on percussion (if a haemothorax is present, hyporesonance might be present).
- Tracheal deviation to the nonaffected side.
- Cardiac arrest.

Treatment

In an emergency, thoracocentesis is performed by competent personnel. This involves placing a large-bore (14G) cannula in the midclavicular line of the second intercostal space to release the pressure. A chest drain should then be inserted.

Cardiac tamponade

Pericardial effusion is an abnormal collection of fluid in the pericardial sac. If this causes haemodynamic comprise it becomes cardiac tamponade. Tamponade usually occurs quite rapidly. If fluid builds up slowly it can be quite well tolerated.

Causes

Cardiac tamponade can be caused by the following:
- Trauma
- Cardiac surgery
- Following pacing wire removal
- During cardiac catheterization
- Malignancy
- Cardiac rupture post MI.

Signs and symptoms

The symptoms include ↑ CVP or JVP, with a further ↑ during inspiration, ↓ BP, SOB, muffled heart sounds, signs of ↓ CO and, occasionally, abdominal pain. In acute cases, e.g. following cardiac surgery, cardiac arrest could occur.

Investigations

- CXR
- ECG—ventricular complexes might be smaller than normal
- Echo.

Treatment

Management depends on the patient's condition. Many patients have pericardial effusions after cardiac surgery that resolve without problems. If an effusion is recurring, a pericardial window might be created. If the patient is severely compromised, pericardiocentesis (needle aspiration) is performed. This should be performed with Echo guidance unless in an emergency cardiac arrest situation. In some cases, a pigtail catheter is inserted that can be left in for up to 24h. If cardiac tamponade has occurred within 48h of cardiac surgery, the patient is usually taken back to the operating theatre for removal of clots and determination of the source of bleeding.

Pulmonary oedema

Pulmonary oedema is a life-threatening emergency. The patient is often very distressed and might feel that they are about to die. The causes of pulmonary oedema include fluid overload and acute MI, and an acute episode might occur in someone who has chronic heart failure. The patient could have the following signs and symptoms:

- ↑ SOB
- Pink or blood-stained, frothy sputum
- Respiratory rate >25 breaths/min
- ↓ SaO_2
- ↓ BP
- Peripheral shutdown
- Tachycardia
- Profuse sweating
- Wheezes and crackles on auscultation.

Investigations

- CXR
- ECG—to exclude STEMI
- SaO_2
- ABG
- Cardiac biomarkers
- FBC, U&E, CRP
- Echo.

Management

Position the patient upright with the support of many pillows. Some patients find sitting in a chair more comfortable. Give 60% humidified O_2 through a mask unless the patient has CO_2 retention. CPAP may also be required. Give IV diamorphine and IV furosemide, which is usually followed by an infusion of furosemide (as prescribed). Antiarrhythmics or DC cardioversion might be needed if the patient has an arrhythmia. K^+ levels should be monitored and corrected, as required. Vasodilators may also be given and an infusion of GTN is often prescribed (if no contraindications). In some cases, inotropic support, such as dobutamine (📖 Inotropes, p.373) might be required. Reperfusion for STEMI. The patient will need a urinary catheter and continuous monitoring of CVS observations, respiratory rate, SpO_2, and urine output.

Cardiogenic shock

Cardiogenic shock is often due to significant and often irreversible damage to the LV and manifests in the following ways:
- Acute circulatory failure
- Arterial hypotension
- ↓ urine output
- ↓ level of consciousness
- Rapid, weak pulse
- Cold and cyanosed extremities.

Cardiogenic shock should be differentiated from any other kind of shock. Causes of cardiogenic shock include the following:
- Acute MI
- PE
- Cardiac tamponade
- Rupture of valve cusps
- Ruptured LV aneurysm.

Signs and symptoms

CO ↓ initially, which leads to a ↓ in urine output and an ↑ in pulse. This triggers mechanisms, such as vasoconstriction, which lead to a ↓ in peripheral perfusion and metabolic acidosis.

Management

Patients should be urgently assessed for suitability for PCI. Invasive monitoring, such as PA, PAWP, and arterial monitoring, is usually required to aid treatment. The patient should be catheterized to monitor urine output closely (aim for 0.5mL/kg of body weight/h). Fluids might need to be given if RV infarction is present (📖 Specific principles for nursing patients with ST-segment elevation ACS, p.126). Opiates, such as IV diamorphine, can help to relieve preload, in addition to pain. Monitor ABG and O_2 saturation levels and give O_2 therapy accordingly. Medical management might include inotropes, IV nitrates, IV vasopressors or, in some cases, an IABP (📖 Intra-aortic balloon pumps (IABPs), p.350) or LVAD (📖 Ventricular assist devices, p.354). Support for the patient and family is vital; the prognosis is often poor.

Intra-aortic balloon pumps (IABPs)

Description

The IABP is a counterpulsation device placed in the aorta, just below the aortic arch (See Fig. 18.7), which deflates and inflates in a controlled manner. The balloon holds ~30–40mL of gas, which is usually either helium or CO_2. The patient's ECG or cardiac cycle triggers inflation and deflation. The balloon can be set to inflate every one, two, three, or four contractions. The IABP has two 1° benefits for the heart, as follows:

* The balloon deflates just before systole and, ∴, ↓ the workload of the heart by ↓ the afterload.
* The balloon inflates in diastole, which ↑ blood flow to the coronary arteries and brain.

2° benefits include improvements in cardiac output, ejection fraction and systemic perfusion and a ↓ in heart rate, PAWP, and systemic vascular resistance.

Indications

The IABP should only be placed in those patients where it is felt there will be an improvement in their condition:

* LVF or cardiogenic shock that is not responding to pharmacological agents.
* Severe pulmonary oedema.
* Acute MR.
* Unstable angina.
* Post cardiac surgery if it has been difficult to take a patient off bypass.
* Pre cardiac surgery in unstable patients.
* A bridge to cardiac transplantation.
* A support during coronary angiogram/angioplasty for unstable patients.

Contraindications

* Aortic insufficiency
* Severe aortoiliac disease
* Aortic dissection
* Prosthetic graft in thoracic aorta
* Irreversible brain damage
* Severe peripheral vascular disease.

(a) Cardiac diastole (b) Cardiac systole

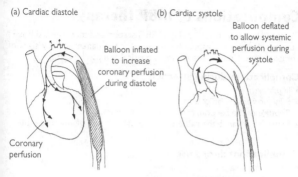

Fig. 18.7 Intra-aortic balloon pump position. Reproduced with permission from Ramrakha P and Moore K (editors) *Oxford Handbook of Acute Medicine.* 2nd edition, 2004. Oxford University Press, Oxford.

Complications of IABP therapy

Complications can occur during IABP insertion and after the IABP is *in situ*. It is the nurse's responsibly to monitor the patient for any signs of complications. Complications can be physical and psychological.

Complications during insertion

- Haemorrhage.
- Puncture/dissection of aorta.
- Rupture of the balloon, causing a gas embolism.
- Failure to advance the catheter far enough because of atherosclerotic disease.

Complications during use

- Limb ischaemia.
- Depression and anxiety.
- Back pain.
- Haemorrhage.
- Aortic dissection.
- Timing problems, leading to inappropriate inflation/deflation. This could then lead to an ↑ in cardiac workload.
- Sepsis.
- Thrombocytopenia.
- Thrombus formation.
- Renal failure.

Nursing care

The nurse must observe the patient for any signs of the listed complications, in addition to understanding how the machine works. The longer the IABP remains in place, the greater the risk of complications such as sepsis or anxiety and depression. The patient must stay flat (can sit to no more than 45°) with the affected limb straight, which can lead to back pain, in addition to complications from immobility. Other nursing care includes the following:

- Monitor cardiovascular observations such as HR, BP, RR, MAP—which should reflect an improvement in the patient's condition. Keep MAP at 70mmHg or above.
- Observe limb for any signs of ischaemia—compare each foot for colour, warmth, sensation, and pedal pulses.
- Check BP in both arms and also radial pulses—report any differences.
- Observe the femoral insertion site for signs of infection, haemorrhage, or haematoma formation.
- Monitor urine output (0.5mL/kg of body weight/h) to ensure that the kidneys are being perfused.
- Check the balloon-assisted trace on the machine (Fig. 18.8) and monitor inflation timings.
- Provide psychological support for both patient and family.
- Monitor the patient for chest pain.
- Care of pressure areas.

- Administer anticoagulants, as prescribed. The patient must be on heparin.
- Report any abnormalities of IABP functioning to the perfusionist and doctor.

The IABP might be removed if there are signs of infection or malfunction. As the patient's condition improves, the timing cycle is ↓. It is usually appropriate to remove the IABP when the inflation ratio is 1:4. The heparin infusion should be stopped first and the ACT should fall to <150s. Firm pressure is applied to the puncture site for approximately 30min.

Reitan catheter pump

The Reitan catheter pump[5] has been developed as an alternative to IABP and is used in select patients in some centres. It has a rotating propeller that sits in the upper part of the descending aorta. Rotation of the propeller results in afterload reduction. It can be used in patients with aortic valve problems.

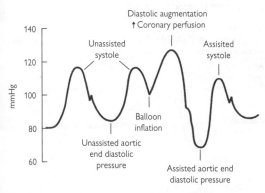

Fig. 18.8 Arterial IABP waveform. Reproduced with permission from Ramrakha P and Hill J *Oxford Handbook of Cardiology*. 2nd edition, 2012. Oxford University Press, Oxford.

---

5 ℐℬ http://www.cardiobridge.com

Ventricular assist devices

Ventricular assist devices (VAD) are used to support the ventricle, improve CO, and ↑ perfusion. They can be used for the left or right ventricle and, in some cases, both ventricles (BiVAD). VAD are normally used either in acute heart failure (e.g. post MI or if there is an inability to wean the patient from cardiopulmonary bypass) or as part of longer-term management in patients with chronic heart failure or cardiomyopathy. Although the risks of thromboembolic complications have ↓ with improvements in the devices, the risk of infection and sepsis is high. It is important that VAD are only used in patients in whom the benefits of the device outweigh the risks. They can be used in the short term, as a bridge to transplantation, or on a longer-term basis.

Devices are extracorporeal or implantable. Various models of VAD are used but all models require an external power source that is connected to the device by drive lines. This can be a portable device or a consul by the bedside. For LVAD, the left atrium or ventricle is connected to the aorta by a pump. For RVAD, the right atrium is connected to the pulmonary trunk. Devices can be set at a fixed rate or set to work if the stroke volume ↓. In all cases, anticoagulation is required, in addition to strict attention to minimizing infection risk. Education and support for both patient and family are extremely important.

Complications

The risk of complications ↑ with the ↑ length of time the device is *in situ*. Complications might include the following:
- Infection
- Thromboembolism
- Psychological problems, such as depression and anxiety
- Bleeding
- ↓ CO
- Kinking of lines
- Rhythm abnormalities.

Extra corporeal membrane oxygenation

Extra corporeal membrane oxygenation (ECMO) is a supportive therapy which has traditionally been used for patients with severe respiratory distress but can also be used in patients with a low CO. It is similar to the heart bypass machine used during cardiac surgery, but can be used for longer. Blood is pumped through a machine that removes CO_2 and adds O_2. Oxygenated blood is then returned to the body. Patients on ECMO will normally be nursed in the ITU.

Types of ECMO

There are two different types of ECMO. Venovenous ECMO (VV) which is used for respiratory support and venoarterial ECMO (VA) for mixed cardiac and respiratory support. In VV ECMO venous cannula are usually placed in the right femoral vein (for removal of blood) and the right internal jugular vein (for returning blood). In VA ECMO the venous cannula is placed in the right femoral vein and the arterial cannula is placed in the femoral artery. The patient would be on a heparin infusion.

Indications for ECMO

Indications for ECMO include the following:
• Hypoxemic respiratory failure unresponsive to ventilator support
• Cardiogenic shock
• Cardiac arrest
• Bridge to cardiac transplantation
• Failure to wean from CPB post cardiac surgery

Ventricular rupture and ventricular septal defects

Congenital VSDS are described in Chapter 14 (📖 Ventricular septal defect, p.279). Post MI some patients develop a VSD or rupture their ventricle. This could lead to cardiogenic shock. An Echo is required to assess the damage and check whether there is any involvement of the heart valves. Surgical repair is usually required. The prognosis is poor in many cases.

Aortic dissection

If a patient develops an aortic dissection, they might present with severe pain similar to that of an MI. This should be excluded. Pain might also be present in their back and abdomen, and it is often described as 'tearing'. The ECG might not show any changes. Causes of aortic dissection include the following:

- Hypertension
- Marfan's syndrome
- ↑ age
- Coarctation of the aorta
- Trauma
- IABP
- Pregnancy.

The location of the dissection influences the associated problems. For example, the renal arteries or aortic valve can be affected. Dissections are classified using the Stanford criteria, as follows (Fig. 18.9):

- Type A—proximal, involving the ascending aorta with or without extension in the descending aorta (2/3 of patients).
- Type B—distal, involving the descending aorta without involvement of ascending aorta.

Signs and symptoms

The patient might be hypotensive (~20%) or have a normal or elevated BP. Other signs and symptoms include the following:

- Severe pain—this might vary according to the type of dissection. If the pain is anterior, it is more likely to be a proximal dissection (Type A). If the pain is towards the patient's back, it is likely to be distal (Type B). It is important to differentiate the pain from STEMI.
- Tachycardia.
- Nausea and vomiting.
- Pale.
- Sweaty.
- Other symptoms depend on the extent of the dissection, e.g. MI, haematuria (if renal artery involvement), CVA, or neurological deficit.
- Different BP recording in each arm.

Investigations

- CXR—↑ width of mediastinum.
- ECG—LVH. This may mimic STEMI as ST elevation may be present.
- TOE.
- CT or MRI scan.

Management

A thorough assessment of the location of pain and associated symptoms is important. This can give clues about the type of management required. Give pain relief (usually IV opioid) and monitor effectiveness. The nurse should perform urinalysis to check for blood and protein and assess neurological status carefully. Record the BP in both arms. Also monitor peripheral perfusion carefully. Hypertension may be managed with either β-blockers or another type of vasodilator, such as sodium nitroprusside. Also provide psychological support. Type A dissections usually require urgent surgery, whereas Type B dissections can be managed medically.

TYPE A   TYPE B

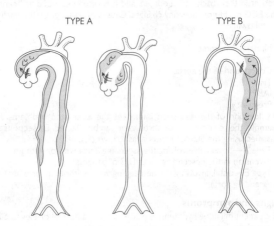

Fig. 18.9 Stanford classification of aortic dissection. Reproduced with permission from Myerson SG, Choudhury RP, and Mitchell ARJ (eds) (2010). *Emergencies in Cardiology* 2nd edn. Oxford University Press, Oxford.

Related guidance

European Society of Cardiology (2008) Guidelines on the diagnosis and management of acute pulmonary embolism. *European Heart Journal* **29**, 2276–315.

National Institute for Health and Clinical Excellence (2010) *Venous Thromboembolism: Reducing the Risk*. NICE, London.

National Institute for Health and Clinical Excellence (2012) *Venous Thromboembolic Diseases: The Management of Venous Thromboembolic Diseases and the Role of Thrombophilia Testing*. NICE, London.

National Institute for Health and Clinical Excellence (2011) *Extracorporeal Membrane Oxygenation for Severe Acute Respiratory Failure in Adults*. NICE, London.

National Institute for Health and Clinical Excellence (2011) *Therapeutic Hypothermia Following Cardiac Arrest*. NICE, London.

Resuscitation Council (2010) *Resuscitation Guidelines*. Resuscitation Council, London

Scottish Intercollegiate Guidelines Network (2010) *Prevention and Management of Venous Thromboembolism*. NHS Quality Improvement Scotland.

Cardiovascular drugs

Introduction

The aim of this chapter is to give the reader a brief overview of the main groups of drugs used in the field of cardiac nursing. For each group of drugs, there is a brief description of why they are used, their mechanism of action, examples commonly used in clinical practice, and nursing considerations.

However, it is important that nurses keep themselves updated in the use of drugs by reading research papers and international, national, and local guidelines. For doses of drugs, methods of administration, contraindications, and side effects, use a recognized formulary, in addition to any local policy.

Antiarrhythmics

Uses

Antiarrhythmic agents are used in the treatment of both supraventricular and ventricular arrhythmias. Some agents are specifically used to treat supraventricular arrhythmias (e.g. verapamil and adenosine), some agents treat ventricular arrhythmias (e.g. lidocaine [lignocaine]) and some agents (e.g. disopyramide and amiodarone) can act on both types of arrhythmia.

Mechanism of action

Antiarrhythmics correct arrhythmias by different mechanisms, and as a result, this group of drugs are generally classified by their mechanism of action on cardiac conduction. Generally, they can suppress arrhythmias by blocking either the action of specific ion channels or the effect of the autonomic nervous system. ∴, knowledge of the cardiac action potential (AP) and the autonomic nervous system assists in understanding their mechanism of action.

Examples

One frequently used classification system is the Vaughan Williams system (Table 19.1). However, some drugs can fit into more than one category (e.g. sotalol), whereas other drugs that are also used as antiarrhythmics are not included. The drugs in the latter category are adenosine, cardiac glycosides, and atropine.

Table 19.1 The Vaughan Williams classification system

Class	Mechanism	Drug
Ia	Sodium-channel blocker (↑ duration of AP)	Procainamide, disopyramide
Ib	Sodium-channel blocker (↓ duration of AP)	Lidocaine (lignocaine)
Ic	Sodium-channel blocker (little effect on duration of AP)	Flecainide, propafenone
II	β-adrenoceptor blockers	Propranolol, sotalol
III	Potassium-channel blocker (prolongs the AP)	Amiodarone, sotalol Dronedarone
IV	Calcium-channel blocker	Verapamil

Advances in the field of pacing, cardioversion, and defibrillation, however, are limiting the role of antiarrhythmics in the clinical setting.
Dronedarone has Class III effects but also Class Ib, IV and II, and is used as a treatment for atrial fibrillation.

Nursing considerations

- Antiarrhythmics can also cause undesired alterations to the rate, rhythm, and contractility of the heart, and they often have many other side effects. It is, ∴, important to monitor patients, particularly HR and K^+ levels.
- A number of other drug groups interact with antiarrhythmics so it is important to check for possible drug interactions. There is an ↑ risk of ventricular arrhythmias with drugs other than those commonly used to manage cardiac conditions, including antimalarials, some tricyclic antidepressants, antihistamines, and antipsychotics.
- The concept of 'half-life'. The half-life of a drug is the time it takes for the drug concentration to be reduced by half. ∴, drugs that are said to have a short half-life, e.g. adenosine (which has a half-life of ~10s), need to be administered frequently and will leave the body quickly. The impact of any side effects is minimal. A drug with a long half-life, e.g. amiodarone (which has a half-life of ~100 days), takes a long time to reach its therapeutic level, so a large loading dose is given, followed by smaller 'maintenance' doses. However, a drug with a long half-life also stays in the body for a long period of time, even after the drug has been stopped. ∴, amiodarone can interact with another drug after it has been stopped a few days, because the circulating levels might still be sufficient to cause an interaction.

There are four classes of antiarrhythmic agent; class 1 is subdivided into three subgroups, depending on the effect of the drug on the AP.

Cardiac glycosides

Uses

The most commonly used cardiac glycoside is digoxin. The drug is most useful in the treatment of SVTs and is used to control the ventricular rate in AF or atrial flutter. It can also be used for the treatment of heart failure.

Mechanism of action

The therapeutic effects of cardiac glycosides are attributable to blockade of the $Na^+/K^+/ATPase$ pump. In AF, it slows the ventricular rate largely by ↓ the sympathetic drive and ↓ conduction across the AV node. Cardiac glycosides ↑ the force of contraction and provide inotropic support. Inhibition of the $Na^+/K^+/ATPase$ pump on the cell membranes of cardiac myocytes results in ↑ intracellular sodium. This ↑ in intracellular sodium inhibits the sodium–calcium exchanger, and thus ↓ the efflux of calcium ions, resulting in an ↑ in intracellular calcium. ↑ intracellular calcium results in ↑ contractility.

Example

Digoxin.

Nursing considerations

- Patients must be monitored for side effects, which fall into two categories: cardiac and noncardiac. Cardiac side effects include bradycardia, (possibly) heart block, and ventricular arrhythmias. To monitor for bradycardia, record the HR before drug administration. If the pulse is <60bpm, withhold the dose until medical staff are consulted. Teach patients taking digoxin at home how to accurately take their own pulse.
- Noncardiac side effects include anorexia, nausea and vomiting, and diarrhoea.
- There could also be neurological side effects such as headaches, drowsiness, and confusion. Can also cause visual disturbances.
- Ensure blood digoxin levels are monitored to prevent toxicity.
- Monitoring of blood potassium levels is very important because hypokalaemia can ↑ the likelihood of digoxin toxicity. ∴, caution must be taken when administering potassium-lowering drugs such as diuretics. Give either potassium-sparing diuretics or potassium supplements.
- Digoxin might need to be stopped before cardiac surgery to ↓ the risk of arrhythmias or bradycardia postoperatively, but check with medical staff. This is because alterations in potassium levels after surgery can cause the effects of digoxin to fluctuate.
- Lower doses may be required for elderly patients as they tend to be more sensitive to the effects of digoxin and are ∴ more likely to experience side effects.

β-blockers

Uses

- Hypertension
- Angina—↓ myocardial workload
- Myocardial infarction—↓ the recurrence rate
- Antiarrhythmic—blocking sympathetic activity
- Heart failure—blocking sympathetic activity
- Anxiety
- Migraine prophylaxis.

Mechanism of action

β-blockers block β-adrenoceptors; these receptors are situated in the heart, bronchi, peripheral vasculature, pancreas, and liver. There are two β-receptor subtypes, which are identified as β_1 and β_2. The β_1 receptor subtype is found in the heart, so blocking these receptors blocks the sympathetic response and, ∴, causes ↓ CO, BP, and HR. However, although some β-blockers are cardioselective, they might also block β_2 receptors. β_2 receptors are found in the lungs and, ∴, a side effect of these agents can be bronchoconstriction. Different β-blockers can be used in different clinical situations.

Examples

Propranolol, atenolol, metoprolol and bisoprolol.

Nursing considerations

- Knowledge of the autonomic nervous system not only enables a good understanding of the mechanism of action of this group of drugs, but it also aids understanding of the side effects, which can include excessive bradycardia, ↓ CO that could predispose some patients to heart failure, and excessive hypotension. ∴, monitor patients carefully so that doses and regimens can be altered to ensure that HR, CO, and BP stay within safe limits. Moreover, a reduction in CO could make a patient feel tired.
- Another very important side effect is bronchoconstriction; ∴, it is not advised that β-blockers (even cardioselective β-blockers) are given to patients with a history of bronchospasm, e.g. asthma and COPD.
- β-blockers can cause peripheral vasoconstriction and patients might suffer from coldness in their fingers and toes. These drugs can have GI side effects, which can be reduced if the drugs are taken before meals.
- Caution should be used when giving β-blockers to patients with diabetes because the signs and symptoms of hypoglycaemia and hyperglycaemia can be masked. ► Monitoring of blood glucose levels is, ∴, important. Patients with diabetes might also need changes to their dose of insulin or oral hypoglycaemics.

- Long-acting β-blockers might need to be stopped before surgery, to ↓ the impact of their effects postoperatively, including bradycardia and ↓ cardiac contractility. Check with medical staff.
- The elderly are more likely to be sensitive to β-blockers and therefore experience more side effects. They may also make the patient less tolerant to cold temperatures.
- One side effect of β-blockers is that they may cause erectile dysfunction. This may impact on the patient's willingness to take the medication and ∴ clear patient education is required.

Calcium-channel blockers

Uses
- Hypertension
- Stable angina
- Antiarrhythmic effects.

Mechanism of action
Calcium-channel blockers ↓ the flow of calcium ions into muscle cells through slow calcium channels of active cell membranes. This calcium blockade occurs in vascular smooth muscle, myocardial cells, and the conduction system. Without calcium, muscles cannot contract, resulting in vasodilation of peripheral and coronary blood vessels, ↓ in myocardial contractility, and a ↓ in the formation and conduction of nerve impulses.

Examples
Within this group of drugs there are the following subgroups:
- Dihydropyridines—e.g. nifedipine and amlodipine, which act predominantly on blood vessels and are, ∴, vasodilators with minimal effect on cardiac activity.
- Nondihydropyridines—which can be subdivided further into verapamil and diltiazem. Verapamil acts on cardiac conduction and is, ∴, administered as an antiarrhythmic. Diltiazem is intermediate between verapamil and the dihydropyridines and has some vascular and cardiac effect.

Nursing considerations
For all drugs that affect HR and BP, it is important to monitor these variables. Because they are vasodilators, patients can initially suffer from flushes and headaches, which should be ↓ over time.
- Calcium-channel blockers ↓ myocardial contractility and can interact with other drugs that ↓ contractility, such as β-blockers and some antiarrhythmics, which could lead to severe haemodynamic deterioration.
- Elderly patients may need to be started on lower doses as they may be more sensitive to this group of drugs than younger patients.
- Verapamil can cause constipation.

Nitrates

Uses

- Prophylaxis and treatment of angina, both stable and unstable.
- IV doses of nitrates are useful in the treatment of acute LVF.

Mechanism of action

Nitrates release nitric oxide in vascular smooth muscle, resulting in relaxation and thus vasodilation. They act predominantly on the venous system, causing venodilation, which ↓ the amount of blood returning to the heart (venous return) and ↓ the preload, thereby ↓ myocardial oxygen demand. There is also some arterial dilation; coronary arteries unaffected by atherosclerotic plaques vasodilate, ↑ the blood supply to the myocardium. Peripheral arterial vasodilation ↓ the resistance against which the heart has to pump.

Examples

Glyceryl trinitrate (GTN), isosorbide dinitrate and mononitrate.

Nursing considerations

- The most common side effects of nitrates are related to vasodilation and include flushes, headaches, and hypotension. Monitor the patient's BP and HR very closely when starting to administer IV nitrates. BP can also drop when nitrates are administered by other routes e.g. S/L or buccal, especially if the patient is not used to taking the drug. Orthostatic (postural) hypotension can also develop when standing, so advise the patient to sit for a few minutes.
- S/L tablets of GTN should not be swallowed because they then become ineffective. ∴ patients should be advised how to take the tablets correctly.
- Tolerance to nitrates can develop, so 4–8h nitrate-free period in every 24h is advised to ↓ tolerance.
- If an attack of angina is unresponsive to a couple of doses of GTN, it could be an MI and immediate medical assistance is required.
- Patients need to be informed that they can take nitrates during an episode of chest pain, but can also do so before starting any activities that are likely to precipitate chest pain e.g. climbing stairs.
- Short-acting GTN tablets should be kept in the container they are dispensed in and closed with a foil-lined cap. Once opened, they should be discarded after 8wks as they lose their effectiveness.

Vasodilator antihypertensive agents

Use
Hypertension.

Mechanism of action
The drugs produce vasodilation of arteries, resulting in a ↓ of peripheral vascular resistance and a consequent ↓ in BP.

Examples
Hydralazine dilates arteries. Sodium nitroprusside, another drug in this group, releases nitric oxide, which relaxes vascular smooth muscle in both arterial and venous systems, ↓ preload and afterload, and resulting in a ↓ in BP.

Nursing considerations
- Hydralazine can cause tachycardia and ↑ fluid retention.
- Sodium nitroprusside has a short duration of action and, ∴, must be administered IV. The drug, however, has poor physical stability so the infusion must be made up regularly and protected from exposure to light. In the presence of light, the drug can be degraded to cyanide. The nurse must, ∴, ensure that all parts of the infusion apparatus are covered.

Angiotensin-converting enzyme inhibitors

Uses
- Cardiac failure.
- Hypertension, particularly in insulin-dependent diabetics
- Management post-MI.

Mechanism of action
ACE inhibitors work on the renin–angiotensin–aldosterone system (RAAS). An understanding of this system enables a more exact understanding of the mechanism of action of this group of drugs. Renin is an enzyme that converts angiotensinogen into angiotensin I; angiotensin I is then converted into angiotensin II in the lungs by ACE. Angiotensin II is a powerful vasoconstrictor and stimulates the release of aldosterone, which ↑ sodium and water retention. So, by blocking the action of ACE, there is vasodilation and a ↓ in fluid volume, leading to a ↓ in BP.

Examples
Captopril, lisinopril, enalapril, ramipril and perindopril.

Nursing considerations
- Within a few hours of administration of an ACE inhibitor, BP can drop. ∴, start these agents at low doses and monitor very carefully.
- Potassium concentrations can rise in patients taking ACE inhibitors, which is important if patients are also taking potassium-sparing diuretics or potassium supplements. Hyperkalaemia can cause arrhythmias.
- One side effect of ACE inhibitors is a persistent dry cough, which can be irritating; the mechanism by which ACE inhibitors cause this side effect is thought to be linked to the accumulation of kinins, which are irritants within the lung.
- ACE inhibitors are associated with a ↓ in renal BP and thus ↓ filtration pressure, so monitor renal function. However, these drugs seem to offer renal protection in diabetic patients.

Angiotensin II antagonists

Use

Hypertension, in particular to ↓ BP in patients who cannot tolerate ACE inhibitors.

Mechanism of action

These agents do not block the conversion of angiotensin I to angiotensin II in the same way that ACE inhibitors do; they block the action of angiotensin II at its receptor site.

Examples

Losartan and candesartan.

Nursing considerations

Monitor the patient as described for ACE inhibitors (📖 Angiotensin-converting enzyme inhibitors, p.371).

Inotropes

Uses

- To ↑ cardiac muscle contractility and to maximize oxygenation of tissues.
- To treat shock.

Mechanism of action

This group of drugs mimic the sympathetic nervous system and, ∴, to varying degrees, ↑ the contractility of the heart, HR, and BP. Inotropes commonly in clinical use include catecholamines or their derivatives. Knowledge of the autonomic nervous system, and adrenoceptors in particular, is important. To understand the subsequent physiological response, it is important to know the location of α_1 and α_2, β_1 and β_2 receptors and their actions when stimulated. Different inotropic agents have different effects on these receptors, they thus cause different responses and so can be used in different clinical situations.

Examples

Adrenaline (epinephrine) has α_1 activity, causing vasodilation at low doses but vasoconstriction at higher doses. The drug acts on β_1 adrenoceptors to ↑ myocardial contractility. It is used, in particular, for anaphylactic shock, acute allergic reactions, and septic shock, in which there is widespread vasodilation; BP can be maintained by vasoconstriction. However, adrenaline causes a ↓ in renal blood flow. It is also used in cardiac arrest.

Noradrenaline (norepinephrine) has similar effects to adrenaline; however, it is a much more potent arterial constrictor agent than adrenaline. The drug is sometimes used to treat acute hypotension, but the intense vasoconstriction must be balanced against ↓ perfusion to the vital organs, especially the kidneys.

Dopamine acts on different receptors, depending on its dose. At low doses, D_1 receptors, which are found in vascular smooth muscle, are stimulated and cause vasodilatation in the renal and mesenteric vascular beds, improving renal blood flow. At the next dose, B_1 receptors are activated, ↑ HR and myocardial contractility, and at higher doses, α adrenoceptors are activated, causing an ↑ in vasoconstriction.

Dobutamine affects both α and β adrenoceptors, but the greater effect is on the β adrenoceptors. It causes an ↑ in myocardial contractility but has only a mild effect on HR; therefore, the drug is used for support in cardiac failure.

Nursing considerations

- Ensure all patients given inotropes have central venous access (due to serious effects of extravasation) and are adequately hydrated. Also carefully monitor the patient, including measurement of CVP, hourly urine output measurements, and invasive BP monitoring.
- Measurement of urine output is very important and as a result patients receiving inotropic medication usually have a urinary catheter *in situ*. This will give an indication of renal function as will regular blood tests for U&E.
- If an adrenaline (epinephrine) or noradrenaline (norepinephrine) infusion is used, it should never be stopped abruptly because of the risk of a sudden collapse of the BP.
- Dopamine and noradrenaline are chemically incompatible with sodium bicarbonate.

Anticoagulants

Uses
Prophylaxis and treatment of DVT, PE, unstable angina, and ACS sometimes in combination with thrombolytics.

Mechanism of action
Anticoagulants suppress the production of fibrin, thereby disrupting the coagulation cascade. They inhibit the formation of new clots but do not dissolve existing clots.

Examples
- Heparin inhibits coagulation by ↑ the action of antithrombin III. This prevents the conversion of prothrombin to thrombin and fibrinogen to fibrin. LMWH, e.g. enoxaparin, are heparin fragments. They ↑ the effect that antithrombin has on factor Xa not on thrombin. They tend to be used instead of unfractionated heparin as the effects are more predictable and do not prolong the activated partial thromboplastin time (APTT).
- Warfarin is an antagonist of vitamin K and inhibits the hepatic manufacture of coagulation factors II, VII, IX, and X.
- Dabigatran is a thrombin inhibitor, so preventing thrombin from enabling the conversion of fibrinogen to fibrin.

Nursing considerations
- Warfarin is only administered orally; in hospital, it is usually administered in the evenings so that the dose can be altered according to the patient's blood test results.
- Heparin is administered by IV or SC infusion.
- Dabigatran is administered orally.
- The two major risks with anticoagulants are as follows:
  - Overanticoagulation, with resultant bleeding. Counteract heparin with protamine sulphate; counteract warfarin with vitamin K. There is no specific drug to counteract dabigatran.
  - Inadequate anticoagulation, leading to the formation of clots.
- Patient education—all patients must be advised to observe for any signs of excessive bleeding and to report this to medical or nursing staff.
- There are many drug interactions with warfarin, which must be checked in a recognized formulary. However, key drug interactions include alcohol and aspirin, which both enhance the effects of warfarin. Patients should also be advised that there may be interactions between warfarin and some herbal products and this should be discussed with their doctor.
- Warfarin is usually stopped 2–3 days before surgery and the patient commenced on heparin; this allows for tighter management of the coagulation profile and quicker reversal of anticoagulation, if necessary. Check with the medical staff.

- Oral anticoagulants are known to be teratogenic and can cause fetal abnormalities in the early stages of pregnancy and fetal haemorrhage in the later stages. ∴, ♀ must inform their doctor if they are pregnant or likely to become pregnant.
- Patients need to be advised that they will need regular blood tests to monitor their clotting profile (INR). The blood tests may be performed in outpatient clinics, although there is ↑ use of home testing kits.

Antiplatelets

Uses

Prevention of MI and cerebrovascular events (such as CVA). (See also
📖 Pharmacological adjuncts to PCI, p.157.)

Mechanism of action

Generally, this group of drugs interferes with platelet membrane function,
prevents release of platelet constituents, and inhibits platelet aggregation.

Examples

- Aspirin, the most commonly used agent, works inside platelets,
  inhibiting the formation of thromboxane A2 from arachidonic acid
  by blocking the enzyme cyclooxygenase (COX). This results in the
  inhibition of platelet aggregation. It is used as 2° prophylaxis.
- Clopidogrel interferes with platelet function by inhibiting adenosine
  diphosphate-mediated platelet aggregation.
- Abciximab is in a group of drugs known as glycoprotein IIb/IIIa (GPIIb/
  IIIa) inhibitors. GPIIb/IIIa receptors on platelets are blocked which
  effectively stops platelet aggregation, this prevents further platelet or
  fibrinogen binding.

Nursing considerations

- Administer oral drugs with food because this improves the absorption
  of ticlopidine and can ↓ the gastric irritation caused by aspirin.
- Monitor the patient for side effects including bleeding disorders,
  nausea, and vomiting.
- Can ↑ the risk of bleeding if given with anticoagulants.
- A single dose of aspirin (150–300mg) is given following an ischaemic
  event. Ensure that the patient and family are aware that the drug is
  being given for its antiplatelet action and not as an analgesic.
- Aspirin might be stopped before surgery to ↓ the probability of
  postoperative bleeding. Check with the medical staff.

Thrombolytics

Uses
- Acute MI
- PE
- CVA.

See 📖 Specific principles for nursing patients with ST-segment elevation ACS, p.126.

Mechanism of action
Also called 'fibrinolytics', their purpose is to break down existing clots. This is achieved by the activation of plasminogen into plasmin. Plasmin is a protease enzyme that breaks down the fibrin matrix of the clot.

Examples
Streptokinase, reteplase, tenecteplase.

Nursing considerations
- Start thrombolytic therapy as soon as possible after diagnosis and elimination of contraindications, which include recent haemorrhage, surgery, severe uncontrolled hypertension, and known hypersensitivity.
- Streptokinase is a protein derived from streptococci bacteria and, ∴, ↑ the risk of an allergic reaction. Antibodies can develop and ↓ the effectiveness of further treatments with this drug. ∴ general advice is not to use streptokinase once used.
- Monitor patient for bleeding and anaphylactic reactions.

Statins

Uses

- Hypercholesterolaemia.
- Hyperlipidaemia in patients who have not responded to diet.
- To slow the progression of atherosclerosis.
- To prevent coronary events.

Mechanism of action

Statins are 3-hydroxy-3-methyglutaryl-coenzyme A (HMG-CoA) reductase inhibitors. HMG-CoA reductase is the rate-determining enzyme in the synthesis of cholesterol. Therefore, if this enzyme is inhibited, less cholesterol is made, especially in the liver. Also ↑ the liver's ability to remove cholesterol.

Examples

Simvastatin, atorvastatin, and pravastatin.

Nursing considerations

- Statins are more effective if taken in the evening, because the HMG-CoA reductase enzyme is most active during the night, which is, ∴, the time cholesterol is made.
- Contraindicated in liver disease and pregnancy.
- Can cause muscle problems ranging from myalgia (pain) to rhabdomyolysis (damaged muscles). Advise patients to report any unexplained muscle pain, weakness, or tenderness.
- Perform LFT before and within 4–12wks of starting statin treatment. This should be reviewed at 6mths and 1yr because altered liver function is a potential side effect of statins.

Diuretics

Uses
Treatment of oedema and hypertension.

Mechanism of action
Diuretics ↑ the volume of urine flow by affecting ion transport in the nephron. The principal sites of action are the proximal convoluted tubule (PCT), thick ascending loop of Henle, distal convoluted tubule (DCT), and collecting duct.

Diuretics are classified according to their mechanism of action. This is important to know because it helps to predict the magnitude of diuresis, the pattern of electrolyte loss and, ∴, side effects.

Examples
Bendroflumethiazide belongs to the class of 'thiazide and related diuretics'. These drugs work at the beginning of the DCT and inhibit sodium reabsorption. If sodium is not reabsorbed, less water is reabsorbed, causing ↑ diuresis. The drugs are moderately effective because most sodium is absorbed before it reaches the DCT. Thiazide-like diuretics are used to treat hypertension and ↓ oedema in heart failure.

Furosemide belongs to the class of 'loop diuretics' because of its site of action. Loop diuretics work primarily by blocking the $Na^+/K^+/2Cl^-$ co-transport system in the thick ascending limb of the loop of Henle. As a result, sodium and chloride reabsorption is inhibited, but that also means that the loss of potassium ions is ↑. These are powerful diuretics because up to 35% of NaCl is reabsorbed at this part of the loop of Henle. These agents are used to treat pulmonary oedema in LVF and also CCF.

Spironolactone and amiloride belong to the class of 'potassium-sparing diuretics', although they have different mechanisms of action. Spironolactone inhibits aldosterone, a hormone produced by the adrenal cortex, which results in not only ↑ excretion of sodium, and ∴ water, but also conservation of potassium. Amiloride primarily works by inhibiting the passage of sodium into the late DCT and collecting duct, thereby preventing the movement of potassium out into the fluid. As a result of their mechanisms of action, they are weak diuretics and are usually given with other diuretics in order to prevent hypokalaemia.

Nursing considerations
- Monitor patients on diuretics; this should include vital signs, weight, and fluid balance. ▶ It is very important to monitor potassium levels, especially in patients who are not taking potassium-sparing diuretics.
- It is important to monitor blood glucose levels closely in diabetic patients because these drugs can cause hyperglycaemia.

- It is advised that patients take diuretics in the morning and the early afternoon to avoid having a disturbed night with frequent episodes of passing urine. Thiazide diuretics have a long duration of action (12–24h) so should be taken in the morning only; however, the action of furosemide only lasts up to 6h so it can be administered twice daily without causing sleep disturbance.
- Furosemide must be administered slowly at a rate not exceeding 4mg/min to prevent ototoxicity, which damages hearing.
- Medical staff might review or stop diuretic use before cardiac surgery to help maintain control over fluid balance and ↓ arrhythmias postoperatively.

Appendix 1

Further suggested resources

This book is intended as a quick reference text, and ∴ I have included some suggestions for further reading and some websites that you might find useful. There is a wealth of available literature on all of the topics covered in this book and it would be impossible to cite all of it here. The following list is by no means exhaustive and I apologise to those authors whose texts I have unintentionally missed.

Journals

- *British Journal of Cardiac Nursing*
- *British Journal of Cardiology*
- *European Heart Journal*
- *European Journal of Cardiovascular Nursing*
- *Journal of Cardiovascular Nursing*.

Books

Albarran J and Tagney J (2007) *Chest Pain: Advanced Assessment and Management Skills*. Blackwell Publishing, Oxford.

Chikwe J, Beddow E, and Glenville B (2006) *Cardiothoracic Surgery*. Oxford University Press, Oxford.

Hatchett R and Thompson D (eds) (2008) *Cardiac Nursing. A Comprehensive Guide* (2nd edn). Churchill Livingstone, Edinburgh.

Humphreys M (2011) *Nursing the Cardiac Patient*. Wiley & Sons, Chichester.

Kucia A and Quinn T (2010) *Acute Cardiac Care: A Practical Guide for Nurses*. Chichester, Wiley-Blackwell.

Myerson SG, Choudhury RP, and Mitchell ARJ (2010) *Emergencies in Cardiology* (2nd edn). Oxford University Press, Oxford

O'Grady E (2007) *A Nurse's Guide to Caring for Cardiac Intervention Patients*. John Wiley and Sons Ltd., Chichester.

Ramrakha P and Hill J (2012) *Oxford Handbook of Cardiology* (2nd edn). Oxford University Press, Oxford.

Thorne, S and Clift P (2009) *Adult Congenital Heart Disease*. Oxford University Press, Oxford

Woods SL, Froelicher ESS, Underhill Motzer S, and Bridges EJ (2010) *Cardiac Nursing* (6th edn). Lippincott Williams & Wilkins, London.

Useful websites

Arrhythmia Alliance: ⅏ http://www.aral.org.uk

Ashley Jolly Sudden Adult Death Trust (SAD UK): ⅏ http://sadsuk.org

British Cardiovascular Society—links to other groups such as British Association of Nursing in Cardiovascular Care and British Association of Cardiovascular Prevention and Rehabilitation can be accessed through this website: ⅏ http://www.bcs.com

British Heart Foundation: ⅏ http://www.bhf.org.uk

British Heart Foundation Statistics Website: ⅏ http://www.heartstats.org

British Heart Valve Society: ⅏ http://www.bhvs.org.uk

Cardiac audit ⅏ http://www.ccad.org.uk

The Cardiomyopathy Association: ⅏ http://www.cardiomyopathy.org

Cochrane Collaboration—a useful website for finding the latest systematic reviews: ⅏ http://www.cochrane.org

Department of Health—a useful site for accessing health policy and guidelines: ⅏ http://www.doh.gov.uk

European Heart Network: ℘ http://www.ehnheart.org
European Society of Cardiology: ℘ http://www.escardio.org
Heart Rhythm UK: ℘ http://www.hruk.org.uk
Marfan Association UK: ℘ http://www.marfan.org.uk
National Heart Forum: ℘ http://www.heartforum.org.uk
National Institute for Cardiac Outcomes and Research: ℘ http://www.ucl.ac.uk/nicor
National Institute for Health and Clinical Excellence: ℘ http://www.nice.org.uk
NHS Heart Improvement Programme: ℘ http://www.improvment.nhs.uk/heart
Resuscitation Council (UK): ℘ http://www.resus.org.uk
Scottish Intercollegiate Guidelines Network: ℘ http://www.sign.ac.uk
Society of Cardiothoracic Surgery: ℘ http://www.scts.org
The Somerville Foundation (previously known as the Grown up Congenital Heart Patients Association): ℘ http://www.thesf.org.uk/
World Heart Federation: ℘ http://www.worldheart.org

Appendix 2

Heart diagrams

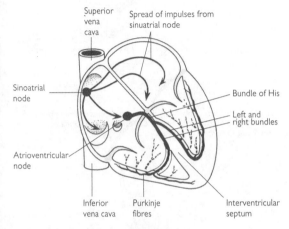

The conduction system of the heart. Adapted with permission from Wilkins R; Cross S; Megson I, and Meredith D. (eds) (2006). *Oxford Handbook of Medical Sciences*, Oxford University Press, Oxford.

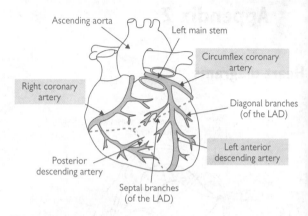

Diagram of coronary circulation. Reproduced with permission from Myerson SG; Choudhury RP, and Mitchell ARJ (eds) (2006). *Emergencies in Cardiology*. Oxford University Press, Oxford.

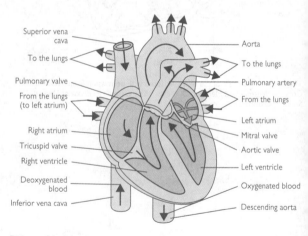

Diagram of the heart

Index